Stepped Care 2.0: A Paradigm Shift in Mental Health

Peter Cornish

Stepped Care 2.0: A Paradigm Shift in Mental Health

Springer

Peter Cornish
Counseling and Psychological Services
University of California
Berkeley, CA, USA

ISBN 978-3-030-48054-7 ISBN 978-3-030-48055-4 (eBook)
https://doi.org/10.1007/978-3-030-48055-4

This Springer imprint is published by the registered company Springer Nature Switzerland AG
The registered company address is: Gewerbestrasse 11, 6330 Cham, Switzerland

Foreword

Once upon a time, mental health services were provided almost exclusively in weekly, 50-min, individual therapy appointments by doctoral-level practitioners operating from their favored theoretical orientations, often with little regard to the research evidence or their patients' preferences. Individual therapy and ideological singularity did not frequently result in salubrious patient outcomes, but did reduce clinical complexity and shared decision-making. And rarely, outside of public health or community circles, did one hear laments about the mountains of underserved or untreated patients. That is not a fairy tale or a clinical dystopia, but the practice paradigm 40+ years ago when I began clinical training.

To be sure, scores of practitioners and researchers in the interim urged care innovations, but those advances largely proved scattered one-trick ponies: add self-help, deliver brief therapy, hire paraprofessionals, conduct more groups, offer e-health and apps, reduce the number of sessions, provide tele-therapy, develop massive open online courses, render only evidence-based treatments, and emphasize population interventions. Meanwhile, the worldwide prevalence of mental disorders rises, wait lists for public care climb, and people continue to suffer. Indeed, according to every reputable metric, the vast majority of people suffering from behavioral disorders do not receive any specialized mental health care at all. At all.

The system is broken, in so many ways. It proves to be inaccessible, inequitable, inefficient, and ineffective (unless you are wealthy and receiving services in the private sector). Everything we have learned in the past four decades tells us that the mental healthcare system has shattered—depriving our patients of responsive treatments, wasting scarce resources, and still neglecting most of those in psychological torment.

Nothing short of a comprehensive and ambitious overhaul is required. *Stepped Care 2.0: A Paradigm Shift in Mental Health* signifies and ignites that overhaul and, in its subtitle's terms, represents a paradigm shift in mental health. You want to improve the care of individual patients and simultaneously enhance the mental health of the entire population? This book provides a strategy and a plan.

SC2.0 features and incorporates so much of what we have learned in recent years about what works and what does not work. It is strength and recovery oriented, not psychopathology consumed. It tailors the intensity of care to the individual, avoiding the prevailing one-size-fits-all. It encourages brief assessments of what actually guides treatment decisions, as opposed to rigid protocols or standard batteries that satisfy administrators. It demands quick and open access to services, not iatrogenic appointments months away or dreaded waiting lists. It is righteously client centric, as opposed to discredited therapist centric. It seamlessly integrates e-mental health and multiple therapy formats instead of replacing or devaluing mental health practitioners. It harnesses the resilience and self-healing of patients, not only the services of professionals. It provides ongoing objective monitoring of outcomes in place of therapist intuition or institutional guesswork. It accommodates the diversity of the population across readiness to change, not only those action-stage treatment seekers. It is population focused, not "one client at a time" as the primary vehicle for improving mental health. It personalizes care, not primarily to diagnoses, but to transdiagnostic characteristics of patient functioning, preferences, and cultures. In short, SC2.0 is a sustainable and systemic restructuring of mental health care.

Its progenitor, the visionary Dr. Peter Cornish, has walked the walk. As a seasoned director of a university counseling center (which I was privileged to visit on two occasions), he battled the growing surge of student-patients and the usual staff resistance to anything more than hiring additional staff. He came to understand that reducing the burden of mental illness necessitates improved access and efficiency in a sustainable manner. He experimented, he failed (forward), he researched, he revised, he researched (more), and eventually he co-developed SC2.0 for the entirety of the Province of Newfoundland and Labrador. He and colleagues have subsequently consulted with more than 100 mental health centers in transforming their services.

A friendly word of warning: If you intend minor tweaking of your mental health services, then this is decidedly not the book for you. You need not agree with every component of SC2.0 (I don't), and you can obviously assimilate parts of the model (I will). But this is a bold, big plan for personalized population health. SC2.0 presents nothing less than innovative disruption in health care, extending the lead of the UK and others.

Their plan and this book are augmented by a dozen training videos demonstrating the model (https://steppedcaretwopoint0.ca/resources/training-videos/) and an interactive PowerPoint presentation (https://steppedcaretwopoint0.ca/interactive-powerpoint/). These will serve as potent introductions to inveterate colleagues and other stakeholders skeptical of anything that challenges their status quo or threatens their treasured proficiency.

The inexorable future of any mature health system will be integrative, universal, responsive care. Using this game-changing text, join Peter Cornish and associates in creating the transformation. As we would say 40+ years ago, be part of the solution!

Department of Psychology
University of Scranton,
Scranton, PA, USA

John C. Norcross

Preface

Origin Story

About 10 years ago, I had to admit that a research project I co-led with a colleague had failed miserably. Rural and remote regions of our province were underserved. This was particularly so for mental health care. Most treatment was provided by either physicians or nurses who admitted feeling unprepared. In an earlier study, we demonstrated some success in providing training and support via distance technology. While this was appreciated, they still did not have the time to focus on mental health treatment. We knew from a literature review that bibliotherapy was effective in treating depression. Would the prescription of an evidence-based self-help text be effective in rural and remote settings? A relatively simple randomized controlled trial would provide the answer. Unfortunately, despite high initial interest expressed by caregivers, we were unable to recruit either healthcare providers or patients for the study. It was a failed study. No worries. Publishing failed studies is important. But the first journal editor disagreed, "Your methodology is flawed, and you should have anticipated the problems." After a few more tries, one editor agreed to publish the work as a commentary if we added more on lessons learned. What did we learn from this failure? The methodology was sound. But the providers told us that they were too busy to give the study full attention. And when they did find time, their patients were not interested. We wondered if the study failed due to a lack of supportive infrastructure. Most sites had only part-time support staff, and they were overworked. Both clinical and support staff were struggling to meet even the basic needs. This was not a methodology problem. It was an infrastructure problem. There were no structures in place to help coordinate or organize treatment, let alone support research. There would need to be a better system in place to support innovation. We became curious about strategies for developing such health system infrastructure. A common lament expressed in the literature is that there is rarely anything systematic about our healthcare system. But surely, there are some system-building success stories. First, I discovered O'Donahue and Drapers 2011 e-book, Stepped Care and e-Health: Practical Applications to Behavioral Disorders (O'Donahue & Draper, 2011). There I was introduced to the stepped care model implemented by the National Health Service in the UK. I was intrigued. Would stepped care for mental health provide the right kind of structure for low-intensity self-help treatments in our rural and remote regions? We offered this as an example of what we might do differently. Sitting on my back deck one morning, feeling pleased with myself as I reread the journal acceptance letter, something clicked. I am the Director of a university counseling center that is struggling to meet demand. Could stepped care help? On that warm summer morning, I quickly sketched out a plan. That sketch was the first of many that eventually led to our nine-step SC2.0 model.

Mental health care is poorly organized. In most places, a help seeker would be lucky to access treatment. There are usually only two options: psychotherapy or psychiatric medication. While undoubtedly effective, demand far exceeds the supply for such specialized programming. Many people seeking to improve their mental health do not need psychiatric medication or sophisticated psychotherapy. A typical help-seeker needs basic support. For knee pain, a nurse or physician might first recommend icing and resting the knee, working to achieve a healthy weight, and introducing low impact exercise before considering specialist care.

Unfortunately, there is no equivalent low-intensity option for mental wellness. As a result, a person seeking the most basic support must line up and wait for the specialist along with those who may have very complex needs. Why are there no lower intensity options? One reason is fear and stigma. A thorough assessment by a specialist is considered best practice. After all, what if we miss signs of suicide or potential harm to others? A reasonable question on the surface; however, the premise is flawed. First, the risk of suicide, or threat to others, for those already seeking care, is low. Second, our technical capacity to predict on these threats is virtually nil. Finally, assessment in our current culture of fear tends to focus more on the identification of deficits (as opposed to functional capacities), leading to overprescription of expensive remedies and lost opportunities for autonomy and self-management. Despite little evidence linking assessment to treatment outcomes, and no evidence supporting our capacity to detect the risk for harm, we persist with lengthy intakes and screens that delay care. Before providers and policy makers can feel comfortable letting go of risk assessment, however, they need to understand the forces underlying the *risk paradigm* that dominates our society and restricts creative solutions for supporting those in need.

In this book, I supply evidence and a plan for dismissing the risk paradigm, freeing providers to extend broadened care options with less caution, thereby ensuring rapid care access for all. It is a realistic plan that can make the work of both help seekers and providers more meaningful, productive, and sustainable.

Stepped Care 2.0 (SC2.0) attends to peoples' capacities, a focus often overlooked when preoccupied with risk. SC2.0 introduces a more balanced approach to assessment and care. It does so in five ways: (1) bringing awareness to the risk paradigm, thereby releasing potential for more creative trial-and-error approaches to wellness; (2) conducting only very brief focused assessment on first contact ensuring time for an intervention; (3) supporting the inclusion of more informal, natural, and community-based healing resources into the traditional circle of care; (4) organizing the increased resources systematically and in a manner that is more readily accessible to all; and (5) continuously adjusting care based on monitoring of functioning, strengths, deficits, risks, and treatment preferences in balance.

SC2.0 reimagines the original UK stepped care model by integrating a range of traditional and emerging online mental health programs systematically within the context of recovery principles and practice. Like the UK approach, SC2.0 offers the lowest level of intervention intensity warranted by objective continuous outcome monitoring. However, unlike the original UK system, which was largely driven by a risk/assessment focus with an emphasis on tracking symptoms (i.e., deficits) and cognitive behavioral therapy approaches aimed at treating the symptoms, SC2.0 allows for the addition of strength-based programming, thus extending the fit to more diverse populations and contexts. This deviation also marks a shift from relying exclusively on *evidence-based practices* derived from controlled experimental conditions. Such a shift is possible with the introduction of *practice-based evidence* using validated measures collected at every encounter with a client. Programming is adjusted based in part on client response and preference rather than relying solely on symptom-based algorithms matched to one-size-fits-all manualized treatment protocols. With this ongoing progress monitoring, practice innovations are encouraged. Program matching decisions in SC2.0 are also more flexible and client centric than in the clinical staging models originally developed in the UK. Rather than stepping only according to diagnosis or symptom severity, one or more options of varying intensity can be jointly selected based on client need, preference, functioning, and readiness for engaging in healing work. Because monitoring is also configured to give both provider and client continuous feedback on progress, the model empowers clients and providers to collaborate more in care options, decisions, and delivery.

As an upstream approach, SC2.0 prevents problems from escalating into serious conditions by systematizing shared responsibility for accessing care options at the right time, with the right people, in the right context. Not only is SC2.0 proving more efficient than traditional mental health service models, early observations suggest that it improves outcomes and access, including the elimination of service wait lists. This book will set the foundation for two subsequent more detailed edited books—one on theory, research, and clinical application and the other on implementation strategies.

Reference

O'Donahue, W. T., & Draper, C. (2011). *Stepped care and e-health: Practical applications to behavioral disorders*. New York: Springer.

Berkeley, CA Peter Cornish

Nobody knows what to do with the electric power of new things.
Heather O'Neall—*The Lonely Hearts Hotel*

Contents

Chapter 1
We Need a Better System

Contents

Crisis What Crisis?
When I was first appointed as the Director of our student wellness centre in 2003, my boss warned she would never support hiring another tenure-track faculty member, even replacements, unless we increased staff productivity. She was true to her word. She disliked the faculty model, arguing that teaching and scholarly duties reduced time available to counsel students. Making matters worse, our clinician-to-student ratio had long been far below average for North American campuses. At the time, faculty would take 1 day per week for research and would be available another day for urgent walk-in client presentations. This was before the surge in demand now commonplace on campuses. The average number of urgent walk-ins per week at the time was no more than 5, meaning we were paying the equivalent of one faculty member to see only one person per day. In 2010, to make better use of this time, all students regardless of urgency were welcome to walk in at any time for an initial appointment. We discovered we did not need crisis counselling as much we thought. What we needed was better access to basic care. And while this change was motivated by a need to increase productivity, it laid the foundation for our current, more client-centric, solution-focused single-session approach.

1.1 System What System?

Interest in mental health has never been higher (American Psychological Association, 2019; Rhydderch et al., 2016). Stigma is decreasing and help-seeking is on the rise (Lipson, Lattie, & Eisenberg, 2018). We have done such a good job with our mental health awareness programs that help-seeking now exceeds the supply of services. Some say we are in the midst of a mental health crisis. This is not the case. What we

P. Cornish, *Stepped Care 2.0: A Paradigm Shift in Mental Health*,
https://doi.org/10.1007/978-3-030-48055-4_1

are facing is a crisis of access. Essentially there are not enough options. A one-size-fits-all approach to mental health care limits options. In Canada, the most accessible care involves consulting a family physician. Unfortunately, family physicians are not well prepared to provide mental health services. Typically, physicians will treat with medication or if that fails, refer to a psychiatrist or psychologist. Wait lists to see both are quite long. Psychologists and psychiatrists are specialists and therefore expensive. Some say just hire more specialists but doing so has limited impact on wait times. Others argue that in order to have meaningful impact we must change how we organize existing programming.

Like many overused words in the English language, the word "system" has become almost meaningless. Too often it is used to describe an incoherent, largely disorganized array of processes or programs. According to the Concise Oxford English Dictionary, the word system is defined as: (1) a set of things working together as parts of a mechanism or an interconnecting network and (2) an organized scheme or method (Soanes & Stevenson, 2008). Most would agree that there is little about mental health care that is interconnected or organized. There is nothing systematic about either our health or mental health care *systems*.

1.2 Neoliberalism in the Context of a Risk Paradigm

In the absence of systems, external socio-political forces drive our care models. In recent decades, neoliberal policies have prioritized global trade, reduced government and increased attention to external threat. The rush to globalize may be slowing, in part due to rising right-wing anti-immigrant populism. These largely unfounded fears further stoke the risk paradigm (Stanford, Rovinelli Heller, & Warner, 2017) that drives news cycles and political agendas.

Socio-political forces have long capitalized on fear to justify hegemonic structures. This is not new. Neither is stoking suspicion to rationalize incarceration of people from the margins of society who might pose challenges to privileged authority. Not long-ago homosexuality was a disease. It was also illegal. Heresy used to be punished by death. Unconventional thinking would lead to asylum confinement. In post-industrial, Eurocentric societies, the marketing of threat has shifted outward to states with emerging economies and cultural traditions that threaten the privileged old-world order. And while domestic terrorism is far more destructive than that of foreign influence, massive risk-industry players continue to drive perceptions of growing external threat. As people drown in limitless, unregulated waves of online information, tribal divisions emerge in efforts to contain the overwhelming barrage. Long gone is the notion of balanced news coverage, once deemed essential for maintaining audience share. In the absence of regulation, cybercrime is on the rise. Risk and surveillance industries, previously the domain of the military–industrial complex, have become the mainstream. These industries depend on perceptions of increasing risk. Stoking risk is essential for growth. A wall, we are told, is needed to keep foreigners out. Cloud-based surveillance systems, we are persuaded, are necessary to protect our homes and communities. We must enable constant streaming, abandoning all rights to privacy, in order to detect all the criminal activity surrounding us.

What do these geopolitical trends have to do with mental health care systems? Fear, stigma and perceived risk have always driven repressive responses to managing mental illness. What is relatively new is the market value attached to a mental health risk paradigm. Over the last 25 years, big pharmaceutical corporations have invested billions in marketing campaigns to convince large segments of the population that normal distress is a biochemical disease. There is very little evidence supporting these claims even for severe and persistent mental illnesses (Greenberg, 2010). Public health messages incorporate this unfounded premise with campaigns urging early detection through mental health screening programs. Airports caution passengers not to leave baggage unattended. Shoes must be removed, and toiletries reduced to micro-doses in carry-on luggage. "See something, say something" signs extend surveillance of odd behaviour to the role civic duty.

When there is extreme and unusually bad behaviour on the scale of a mass shooting, politicians cannot resist temptations to conflate these rare acts of violence with untreated or undiagnosed mental illnesses. There is not a shred of evidence to support these causal links (Varshney, Mahapatra, Krishnan, & Sinha Deb, 2016). There is also no evidence for predicting bad behaviour through psychological or psychiatric assessment (Fazel, Singh, Doll, & Grann, 2012). If the experts can't do it, if there is no convincing relationship between violence and mental illness and there is really no evidence suggesting distress can evolve into a biochemical disease, how are these myths sustained? The answer: they are convenient myths. They distract attention from the real causes of distress and strife.

Journalist Johann Hari suggests the real causes of depression are lost connections (Hari, 2018). He means real connections, not manufactured or commodified ones. False needs are marketed to sell contrived solutions. Forming true social connections takes work and comes with risks. Needs are sometimes stoked, subtly, with fear by creating the perception of risk. Bad breath was not considered a social problem until a mouthwash was marketed. Social anxiety used to be called shyness. Being shy wasn't so bad, but the word anxiety elevates it to the level of disease ripe for social judgement. Normal distress should be prevented or eliminated rather than commodified. The medicalization of distress replaces natural, affirming connections with technical ones. Social media reward mechanisms, such as badges, alerts and scorecards, thereby transforming social interaction into addictive games designed to lure users back to heavily advertised platforms that sell more false needs. More expensive education, the emergence of the gig economy, and continued growing aspirations for soaring lifestyles with houses and vehicles, well equipped with expensive electronics, have increased pressure for students to compete for high-earning careers that may not be personally meaningful. Without connection to purpose, mental health deteriorates. Needs are manufactured to drive addictive, ultimately unfulfilling debt-ridden consumerism. A new gadget, a new outfit or winning the lottery will supposedly bring happiness. But real people, and especially strangers, are dangerous. Social media feels safe because we don't have to leave locked homes where danger lurks behind every bush and in every shadow. Foreigners are either rapists or terrorists. But your own tribe is safe. These are convenient myths that drive our economy and erode our mental health.

The myth of risk is pervasive. The chances of children being abducted by strangers are about 1 in 14 million (Dalley & Ruscoe, 2003). Statistically, strangers are not dangerous. Neither are immigrants. Life expectancy is increasing through much of the world. Poverty, crime and even terrorism are on the decline. Suicide rates are relatively stable with ups and downs commonplace. There is a current upward trend in the United States (Hedegaard, Curtin, & Warner, 2018), but rates were higher in the early twentieth century, the 1930s and the 1990s (Joint Economic Committee, 2019; Efflin, 2019). There are less fatalities from war now than there ever have been (Our World in Data, 2019). For large corporations, this is an inconvenient truth. For Al Gore and the rest of us, the most serious inconvenient truth stems from climate change. Perhaps if we found more ways to connect with nature, that connection would encourage more political action. Even if it didn't, connection to nature is crucial to mental health. It facilitates connection to something larger than us. It allows us to know our purpose, our limits and to fully embrace our short lives.

This disintegration of connections, as it relates to tightening risk management policies, can be seen clearly on university campuses. In the early 2000s, Memorial University of Newfoundland engaged a consulting firm to advise on campus safety. The consultants highlighted unacceptable potential risks associated with the long-standing drinking culture in campus residences. Specifically, student-run residence-life events were targeted for explicitly endorsing binge drinking and social activities that put students at risk, especially female students. The student governance structures were dismantled and stricter policies on consumption of alcohol and drugs were enforced through a new student code of conduct policy. Attempts were made to build identity around academic themes through the development of living learning communities. Health and safety training of residence assistants were expanded, including 2 days of mental health first aid training. The assumption was that through these deliberate well-intentioned student development programs, residence life would mature in alignment with the academic mission of the University. While risky behaviour associated with substance abuse decreased *on campus*, it increased off campus especially in the downtown area about 5 km from the university. In effect, the risk was higher since now students were left with the task of travelling the distance while under the influence.

A set of new modern residence towers opened about 5 years later. In the third week of March of that year—the second to last week of classes of the term—tragedy struck. A female student was found dead by hanging in her residence room shower on Friday morning. In accordance with the postvention protocol of the time, emotional support was offered on site to students and student staff. The multipurpose room on the ground floor was identified as a gathering spot; counsellors were asked to attend along with chaplains and other student affairs staff. Refreshments were served. A decision was made to keep the space open and staff it for 72 h over the weekend. One staff member brought in board games; another brought colouring books. On Saturday, therapy dogs arrived. There were, of course, a lot of tears and hugs among students. The student affairs staff, counsellors and chaplains kept the refreshments supplied but much of the time they clustered awkwardly in the corners sometimes chatting among themselves. The students did not appear to need them. In a review of the procedures the next week, staff and management agreed that the vigil had been longer than it needed to be and that a more rapid return to normalcy would be have been more appropriate. It was unclear how helpful or productive the postvention efforts had been.

As the anniversary of the death in residence drew closer, memories of the previous year resurfaced. Understandably, the mental health first aid training provided over the year had focused more intensively on suicide prevention. Students were anxious about missing the signs but told themselves that increased efforts at identifying students of concern, referring them for help, and in some cases reporting these concerns to more senior residence staff, had made the residence safer. But on the third weekend of March, another female student on the same floor of the same tower, died by suicide in her shower stall.

In discussions with campus leaders following this second suicide we wondered what else we could have done to prevent the deaths. Why had the second one occurred, exactly 1 year later, on the same floor? Did we need to adapt or improve the training protocols? On the one hand, we acknowledged that the rate of suicide on campus over the long run was much lower than in the surrounding city. On the other hand, could this be a new worrying trend? Was it a matter of contagion? We were perplexed and unsettled.

I recall a conversation I had with a senior residence student leader late Saturday evening when we're winding down the postvention support program. As was the case a year earlier, it had been hosted in the multipurpose room on the ground floor of the tower. I asked this student how the room was typically used. He said that it wasn't used much. I wondered why it couldn't be used for something fun or entertaining. After all, games and puppies had been brought in for the postvention session. Why wasn't support, and some kind of positive community engagement the norm? I made a note to myself to consider ways to adjust or expand our clinic-based stepped care model to encourage more social engagement on campus.

1.3 The Original Stepped Care Model

Stepped care is a term that has been used to describe the mental health system developed in the United Kingdom over the past 20 years (Clark et al., 2009). The goals of stepped care are to reduce the burden of mental illness in society and develop a program of care that is self-corrective. To reduce the burden of mental illness, outcomes, access and efficiency need to be increased in a sustainable manner. Typically, the most effective yet least resource-intensive programming is offered first. Programming intensity is only stepped up to the next level with evidence or prediction of failure. Several assumptions drive this stepped care approach. One is that our current system is inefficient with its over-reliance on specialist interventions, including psychotherapy or ongoing psychopharmacological treatment. Both forms of care are expensive, typically offered only by doctoral-level psychologists or psychiatrists. While few would dispute their effectiveness, proponents of stepped care call for the addition of viable lower intensity, less costly alternatives. A second assumption pertains to fit. Traditional care models assume that either psychotherapy or drug therapy will work for everyone. We would not be satisfied with only one or two options for treating physical illnesses. The third assumption is that stepped care achieves efficiencies through a mechanism of self-correction. Care intensity can be stepped up if initial low-intensity interventions fail. Ongoing objective monitoring of outcomes informs stepping decisions in both directions. For example, care intensity can be stepped down following stabilization or after a major reduction in symptom levels.

The original UK approach is referred to variously as a staging, stratified or pathways design (Scott & Henry, 2017). While the evidence supporting staging versions of Stepped Care is mixed, results of clinical trials tend to favour stepped care over treatment as usual (Firth, Barkham, & Kellett, 2015). Extensive up-front assessment is used to stage patients at the appropriate step level. Patients are typically staged according to their symptom levels (see Fig. 1.1). They are referred through corresponding treatment pathways designed to fit symptom profiles. Higher steps of care are offered to people with more severe symptoms, whereas lower steps of care are recommended only for those with mild or moderate symptoms. Staging models assume that symptom levels are a good predictor of treatment outcomes. More specifically, they assume those with severe symptoms would do better with intensive treatment or that people with mild or moderate symptoms will respond best to low-intensity programs. Staging models further assume that people with severe symptoms are more vulnerable and that more vulnerable people need more intensive mental health care. As such, more effort and expense should be targeted at those with higher symptom levels. The assumptions seem logical, however with closer

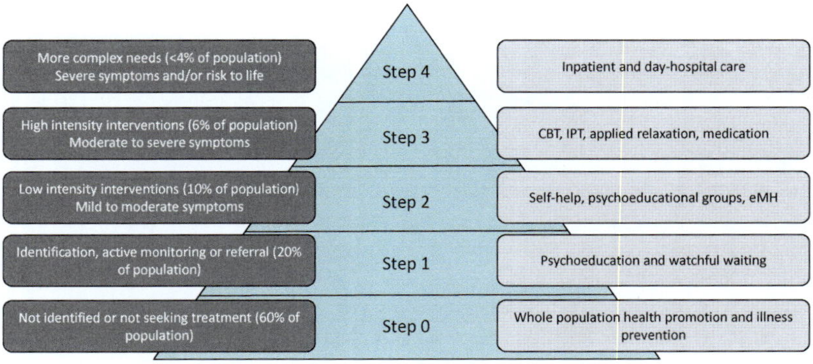

Fig. 1.1 UK-based stepped care staging model. Adapted with permission from (NICE, 2011)

scrutiny, questions arise. What happens when someone with high symptom levels is functioning quite well and is not interested in treatment? And if not ready to engage in treatment despite both low functioning and high symptoms, does it make sense to offer high intensity, expensive care? Or would it be more sensible to support a person with moderate symptoms, low functioning and high readiness to engage? Staging models further assume that people with severe symptoms would not likely benefit from low-intensity treatment. Does this mean peer support would not be offered? Studies suggest that low-intensity e-mental health programs work for people regardless of symptom severity (Bower et al., 2013). While well-intentioned, there is little evidence to justify staging people to treatment pathways based on symptom levels alone.

1.4 What Is Different About SC2.0?

SC2.0 is not a clinical staging model. We do not make step decisions based on symptom severity or complexity. Instead, it is better described as a flexible progressive model. Progressive models offer low intensity first no matter the symptom severity or clinical complexity. A recent study indicated that clients are 1.5 times more likely to recover through a progressive design (Boyd, Baker, & Reilly, 2019). There is growing evidence for considering other variables in treatment planning (Wampold & Imel, 2015). For example, someone with severe symptoms might be highly functional and may not need to be under the care specialist. A motivated, high-functioning person with severe symptoms might wish to direct their own healing process. And even highly symptomatic people with restricted functioning in some areas of their lives might be highly productive in others. For example, a person in the midst of a psychotic break might still be highly sociable and benefit from ongoing support from a peer helper. A simplistic clinical staging model based on only deficit assessment could miss opportunities for supporting recovery.

So, what is different about SC2.0? For one, it is a collaborative model, drawing on recovery-oriented principles to promote client responsibility, autonomy and resilience. In short, it is more client-centric than the staging model of stepped care. SC2.0 starts simple with a focus on people's self-reported issues, goals and capacities. Investigation of potential underlying deficits or pathology is considered only if this strengths-based approach fails to achieve results.

SC2.0 offers a system for developing, adjusting, delivering and monitoring recovery-oriented programs, while promoting client responsibility, autonomy and resilience. Step levels of treatment are based in part on readiness for change. This recognizes that people seeking help are at various stages of readiness to assume responsibility for making the kinds of changes in their lives that will contribute to recovery. For example, some people with intense symptoms of social anxiety may not feel comfortable attending group therapy even though the exposure method is a proven highly effective method for achieving reliable stable and long-term improvements in social functioning. Instead, a person with social anxiety might prefer doing preparation work online, learning about the nature, causes and varied treatment options, before considering exposure as an option. On the other hand, a highly motivated person might be ready and eager to leap right into exposure by attending a public speaking class or social anxiety therapy group.

SC2.0 is more client-centric than staging models. Client centricity is different from being client-centred. Client-centred approaches adapt care to the unique needs of the help-seeker. It eschews a one-size-fits-all all approach to treatment. Client-*centric* care goes one step further. In addition to considering unique needs, client-centric care incorporates client preference and prioritizes client decision-making power. The provider is responsible for outlining the differences in the treatment options, including both what the client might expect from each option and what might be expected from the client in order to ensure success. Once this information is made available, the client decides.

Consider a buffet at a restaurant. If the buffet were client-centric, a patron at the restaurant would have all they need in order to inform healthy choices. This would include adequate description of ingredients. For a commonplace food, a simple label would suffice. For an unusual offering, a more detailed description would be helpful. Foods containing meat, or those designated either gluten or dairy-free would be labelled as such. And of course, staff would be available to address any questions or special needs. An especially spicy food would be marked accordingly. A curry label might include four pepper icons, signalling spicy heat. A patron with sensitivity to spices might recall memories of burning lips or subsequent digestive distress and avoid all of the chili icons. The buffet would include enough information to allow a patron-centric choice.

How might this look at a mental health clinic? A client-centric system is driven more by *informed* preference than symptom severity or treatment intensity. An informed preference is one based on accurate information. This information must specify enough details to ensure informed choices. This would include what can be expected from the product or service, as well what would be expected of the person selecting it.

Let's imagine a client who presents with social anxiety. The discussion of options would include low-, mid- and high-intensity treatments. Low-intensity treatments would require less energy and investment. Mid-intensity treatments might require moderate amount effort, whereas high-intensity treatment would require a high level of commitment, time and energy. At the low end, help-seekers might simply wish to browse the options, learn more about the problem and the potential solutions. There are less urgency and considerable autonomy. At the high end, in contrast, help-seekers would feel more urgency, or be perceived by others as requiring assertive care. The person might be in crisis and incapable of consenting to treatment. The cost in terms of autonomy to the person would be high, treatment might require more time commitment and it could end up being labour-intensive for providers. Alternatively, a stabilizing client-centric treatment plan might rely mostly on involvement of peers or family members. Flexible assertive community treatment team members often include highly capable peer supporters and family members. The team might decide that family support, combined with peer coaching on a mid-intensity e-mental health program is the best option for stabilizing a client.

At the mid-intensity levels, client-centric stepped care might involve a blend of self-help, guided self-help or group programming. While many experts would consider group treatment to be the treatment of choice for someone suffering from social anxiety, such a prescription is likely to be met with resistance by someone who fears social connection. Is it fair to call this resistance? Or would it be more accurate to view it as a natural side effect of an excessive treatment dose? Within the SC2.0 context, several options would be made available to someone interested in working on social anxiety. The lowest intensity option might simply include information about social anxiety delivered online. This could be attractive for someone suffering from extreme social anxiety and not ready for exposure to either a provider or to peers. For someone who is prepared to work with a provider, a guided e-mental health treatment might be tolerable. This combination includes a little exposure in the form of coaching and support, but the e-mental health coursework—the learning—could take place in private at home.

Preference in SC2.0 extends to access modality both for initial contact and ongoing support. Access is possible through a web portal which contains a directory of programming and direct access to a suite of e-mental health programming. Access is also possible through phone (audio and text). Finally, same-day access is possible through local drop-in clinics. While some assessment is conducted at the initial point of contact, the emphasis is on support and care. Many people find the initial contact helpful and seek no further support. For those looking for more, options along the nine-step care continuum can be explored. While models of stepped care vary in terms of the breakdown of steps, nine appears to be the most granular representation (Berger, Fernando, & Salmon, 2020). Our SC2.0 nine-step model is outlined in Fig. 1.2. As steps increase, stakeholder investment (i.e., time, effort, cost to both service users and funders) also increases. Service user autonomy is greatest for lower steps and lowest for high steps.

In contrast to staging models, SC2.0 encourages clients to start with their strengths, to start strong and to start simple. It does this in two ways. First, by drawing on capacities and trusting clients to determine what they wish to focus on, initial goals are manageable. There is no need to identify all the things that may be problematic in a person's life, or a long list of what may be wrong with them. Instead, the approach is simple. What is the thing that concerns you today? What is it that you would like to have changed today as a result of this visit? We don't have to turn over every stone and find what might be wriggling beneath. We don't need to see all the ugly flaws, at least not initially. We start with where the help-seeker is. What interests the person in front of us? What do they want to talk about and what kinds of solutions do they envision? If no solutions are readily at hand, we can dive a bit deeper, turn over a stone or two. But only if necessary.

We acknowledge that we may get it wrong the first time and are transparent about this. It is similar to a visit to a physician. The top of mind concern is briefly assessed and addressed. Follow up is encouraged in the unlikely event the solution fails—"If you are not feeling better in 3–5 days, come back". We make ourselves just as accessible for follow-ups as we do for initial contacts. Unless we are mystified, unless there is something doesn't add up, the simplest solution is likely the best

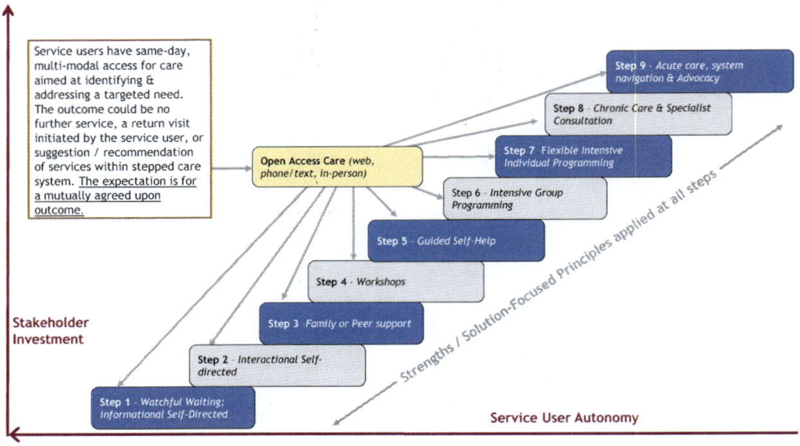

Fig. 1.2 Stepped care 2.0 graphic representation

place to start. We start with Occam's razor—the simple explanation, with further investigation only as needed.

In order to implement this *start-strong/start-simple* approach safely, establishing alignment happens fast. The therapeutic relationship has long been held central to good treatment outcomes. But, of course, it is not the same as a loving marriage. Our goal is not to create a deep attachment. Instead, we work very quickly on setting a trusting working alignment. One way to do this is to take some therapeutic risks. We do this by saying at the outset: "I want to work really hard at developing solutions right now, right here today. I want you to walk away saying 'this was worth my while'.. I also want you to know that I may get it wrong. I need you to let me know if this is the case. At the end of our meeting today, I will give you my card with my email address on it. Let me know if you want to follow up. You can email me, make an appointment or come to the drop-in. If today's work needs some adjustment or rethinking, I'm counting on you to let me know so we can work on it together".

This shared responsibility for trial and error, for building alignment, for taking risks, allows trust to develop quickly. In contrast, a more traditional risk-management approach does the opposite. If the all the interviewer does is ask pre-prepared questions and invests little else in a first encounter, including no attempt at providing care, eliciting collaboration, risking some vulnerability, why would a help-seeker trust the interviewer? For this approach to work, providers need to ensure structures are in place that allows for flexibility and follow-up. Policies and procedures must also support it. Requirements for lengthy screening protocols need to be abolished. Record-keeping content may need adjustments and scheduling processes re-examined. Support for more flexible forms of communication that maintain safety and privacy will need to be in place. Risk managers will have to be convinced of its value. They will need to understand how the empowerment approach shares risk thereby reducing it. They may need help understanding how trial and error is safe.

Communications experts can help reset expectations for and of all stakeholders by promoting, with the right timing and the right audience, how this system is both safer and more empowering. They can help translate the concept of *fail forward* using language that challenges the risk paradigm in a way people are ready to hear. Finding a method to communicate, with sensitivity, the value of failure both in life and academic pursuits, especially for those who are vulnerable already, is no easy task. No one can learn or grow without first being confused or engaged in struggle. Without one or the other, there is no learning or growth. The absence of struggle means either growth didn't happen or wasn't needed. Bold, hopeful, yet sensitive messaging on the new model is an ethical imperative. Shifting expectations with an encouraging voice is crucial for facilitating access and informed consent.

Based as it is in part on the person's readiness to accept challenges, SC2.0 arranges treatments along a continuum of readiness. For example, if a person is looking for support, a listening ear, a place to vent, but is not ready to learn or to develop skills, then a course of intensive psychotherapy would not typically be offered. Instead, less-intensive options are considered. Perhaps connection to a peer support network would be most appropriate. If one-on-one support with some professional oversight is preferred, a clinical trainee could be the best option. Both peer supporters and junior trainees are expected to restrict their interventions to supportive and active listening. This is perfect for a help-seeker not ready to introspect or be challenged. In contrast, for someone who is eager to dig deep and have defences challenged, a course of intensive psychotherapy with a highly skilled therapist would be appropriate.

Client readiness is the third dimension on the SC2.0 continuum. Treatment intensity increases with step level. In order to fully engage with this increasing intensity, clients must be ready for the work and, in the case of the highest steps, to forgo some autonomy. The three dimensions of SC2.0 are illustrated in Fig. 1.3.

Some of my psychotherapist colleagues insist that it is the responsibility of every skilled therapist to apply motivational interviewing. It is a big part of the job to nudge people to full readiness. This seems reasonable. The value of motivational interviewing is well documented (Rubak, Sandbaek, Laurtzen, & Christensen, 2005). However, employing a specialist to do this work is unnecessary. Furthermore, the "nudge to readiness" premise could prove false. Should we always draw *them* to readiness? Or are there times when *we* should move? Maybe we should step back to where they are at the moment. Instead of spending weeks using motivational interviewing to shift readiness, why not shift the treatment intensity and approach to meet the person right where they are?

I can hear my colleagues protest: "What if a person really needs intensive therapy to recover? Shouldn't we do our best to get them prepared for this?" Possibly, but who should decide? And if so, who should we get to do the *horse whispering*? Does this preparatory work need to involve our most highly trained (expensive) specialists? Not likely, but again this could be a joint client–provider discussion focused on preference and expedience. Do we as experts really know what is best for another? What if we are wrong? Why not simply identify what the person is already prepared to do and see what happens? Maybe that would be enough to allow

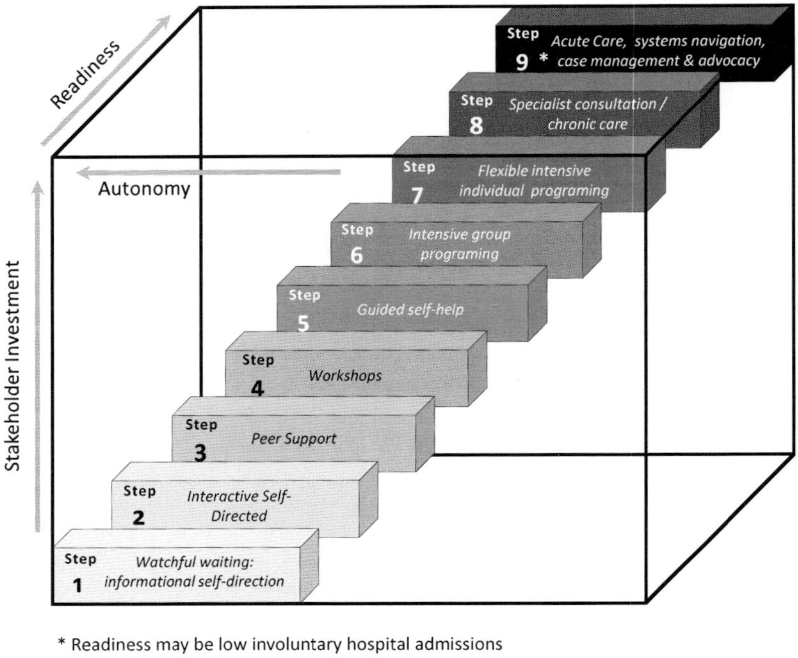

Fig. 1.3 from PowerPoint here

functioning and mental health to recover. If not, the provider and help-seeker can return to the drawing board and fail forward together.

SC2.0 is firmly rooted in recovery principles. Recovery-oriented care assumes that illness and functioning are largely independent dimensions. A person may be mentally ill *and* highly functional just as a person might not be mentally ill and functioning poorly. A recovery model considers more than a person's symptoms or deficits. When it comes to assessment, a recovery model invites us to attend as much to a person's capacities as to their deficits. It also invites practitioners to draw heavily on the expertise of health-seekers. This is not to say a help-seeker has all the answers. But they may be experts on where to begin. They know the top of mind concern. They also know best what they are ready to work on. With SC2.0, we start by believing in capacities and strengths. We have faith in a client's capacity to name the issue they are most ready to work on. With the application of solution-focused interview techniques, often the client comes up with the solution. A single, simple solution co-constructed from the help-seeker's self-identified issue may be enough to stimulate movement to recovery. If not, follow up is easy. Simple is the default.

There can be a few more tries at simple, unless it becomes obvious that simple will not be enough.

My original training looked very different. It was expert-driven. The assumption was, if I was thoroughly trained on psychopathology, diagnostic processes and interventions tied to diagnoses, I would be well equipped to provide the right treatment for the presenting concern. Certainly, this approach is well-intentioned, logical and principled. However, there are a number of fundamental flaws. Diagnostic accuracy is little better than chance. And even when accurate, diagnoses do not inform successful treatment. Neither diagnosis nor technique relates much to outcome. A third problem is that quite often care is delayed by lengthy intake or screening protocols. This lag means lost opportunity. It can contribute to treatment drop out. Imagine a visit to your physician's office for what appears to be an infection. The physician takes the patient's complaint at face value. A full physical is not conducted. The hypothesis that there is an infection is tested in a simple fashion. If confirmed by a brief examination, an antibiotic is prescribed. There was no full physical, or referral for lab tests. Unless something peculiar arises in the investigation the simple hypothesis holds. But of course, the diagnosis could be wrong. It doesn't have to be right. In fact, the physician is quite transparent about failure: "If after 3 or 4 days, you are not feeling better, or if it gets worse, come back to see me". This is recovery-oriented. With SC2.0 mental health professionals begin this way too.

Similar to primary care, SC2.0 begins with targeted brief assessment. And it always identifies strengths. After a question like "What concern is top of mind today", the focus shifts to goal setting. What would you like to be different by the end of our meeting? Or if the issue were to be resolved in the next half hour, what would be different? Have you encountered the issue before? If yes, how did you deal with it? Would that strategy work now? There is no need to reinvent the wheel if we can draw on past successes. We are transparent about the starting strong starting simple approach. And we give options. Are you more interested in exploring what led to this problem or would you rather focus on finding a solution? Whatever the choice, we make clear that this requires a trial and error mentality. I will keep checking in with you to see if we are on track with what is most important to you and we can change course if needed.

Every encounter in SC2.0 is treated as if it may be the last. The goal is to maximize impact because whether we like it or not, a large proportion of visits to providers for mental health concerns are one-time visits. Because the stakes are high, we work to get the most out of every encounter. One way we do this is to infuse each meeting with hope and a conviction that something positive can come out of the session. If we work hard together today on this problem, what is something positive that will come out of it—what we will see at the end of our meeting? Whether or not something concrete is named, the question itself promotes optimism. It also leaves room for failing forward should initial solutions fall flat. I often say we will have about 45 min or an hour today in which I think we can come up something that is helpful. I believe you will leave saying that that was worth my time. It is also possible, I say, that following our meeting today, or maybe tomorrow, you may find yourself concluding that we haven't quite solved the issue yet. I say this is understandable since we only just met. Getting it wrong the first time is no big deal. We can always take another crack at it.

At every encounter, whether through a web portal, by text, over the phone or in person, help-seekers can see the entire buffet of options—all the programming at all the steps. Clients also see their progress reports, the patterns of growth or deterioration and are encouraged to consider, when appropriate the options from the menu that may support continued success or a change of course.

People with lived experience with mental illness have told us formally and informally that they like this model. They are particularly pleased with the straightforward, rapid access to basic care. My colleagues and I initially underestimated the power of same-day access. We thought this might only be relevant to the worried well—those people not at risk but want life to be better. We were wrong, as we learned from the voices of a tiny but resilient community. Like many along the rugged coast of Newfoundland and Labrador, inhabitants are resilient. They have clung to the isolated, storm-ravaged, craggy edge of the continent for almost 500 years.

Everybody Gets Priority

Like much of the coastline in Canada's most easterly province, the scenery on the Burin Peninsula in Newfoundland and Labrador is breathtaking. The population is sparse, strung out long coastal roads that snake along the rocky cliffs, sandy beaches and in and out of the deep protected harbours. But over the course of 16 months in 2016 and 2017 these tiny, sleepy communities were rocked by 14 suicides. In the town of Burin alone, population just over 2000, there were six suicides. Not surprisingly the unusually high numbers of deaths drew national attention. Senior officials from the Government of Newfoundland and Labrador and the Mental Health Commission of Canada visited the region to investigate and deploy resources aimed at preventing further deaths. Initially the plan was to increase resources aimed at identifying those at risk of suicide and targeting services for those who appeared most seriously ill. But members of the community had other ideas. Sisters Natalie Randall and Valerie Peach of the town of Grand Bank both lost their husbands to suicide in 2016. Racked with grief, sadness and anger, Natalie told a reporter that "this Province has to wake up". Both sisters decided to speak publicly to raise awareness of the unmet mental health needs in their region and across the Province. "A culture change is needed" they said because the system is broken with long waitlists and no services at all in many communities. Natalie helped organize a local community mental health coalition in Grand Bank to advocate for change. Organizing for change was also happening in other parts of the Province. The Community Coalition for Mental Health began lobbying the Provincial government in 2015. This led to an unprecedented all-party report recommending dramatic changes structure of the system and delivery of care. The deaths in the Burin region strengthened the resolve of advocates and the all-party committee to seek bold changes.

Rather than demanding more specialist care aimed only at those already ill, community members focused on obtaining rapid access to more basic mental care for the entire population. The best suicide prevention strategy, they argued, is basic, upstream care for all. The Province's Department of Health and Community Services worked closely with members of the coalition and other persons with lived experience to redesign care. One feature of the new system was Doorways, a single session walk-in clinic. The Department had been preparing to establish these clinics province-wide, but at the request of Burin community members, the launch was fast-tracked for their community. Burin community members took the Doorways walk-in concept a step further. The concept of walk-in access was so attractive that they suggested all appointment-based services be transformed immediately to walk-ins. Initially, clinical staff were hesitant as they could not see how all programming could be accommodated through same day access. The coalition persisted and in a matter of months, the wait-list was eliminated, no referrals or appointments were necessary, programming became more client-centric, no-shows and cancelations became a thing of the past. Counselling was available 9–3:30, Monday through Friday at two clinic sites. As one social worker put it, "Everyone gets priority now… not just clients in crisis".

References

American Psychological Association. (2019). *Survey: Americans becoming more open about mental health.* Washington: American Psychological Association. Retrieved January 2, 2020, from https://www.apa.org/news/press/releases/2019/05/mental-health-survey

Berger, M., Fernando, S., & Salmon, A. (2020). *Scoping review of stepped care interventions for mental health service delivery to youth and young adults*. Vancouver: Centre for Health Evaluation and Outcome Sciences.

Bower, P., Kontopantelis, E., Sutton, A., Kendrick, T., Richards, D. A., Gilbody, S., … Andersson, G. (2013). Influence of initial severity of depression on effectiveness of low intensity interventions: Meta-analysis of individual patient data. *BMH, 346*, 1–11.

Boyd, L., Baker, E., & Reilly, J. (2019). Impact of a progressive stepped care approach in an improving access to psychological therapies service: An observational study. *PLoS ONE, 14*(4). https://doi.org/10.1371/journal

Clark, D. M., Layard, R., Smithies, R., Richards, D. A., Suckling, R., & Wright, B. (2009). Improving access to psychological therapy: Initial evaluation of two UK demonstration sites. *Behaviour Research and Therapy, 47*(11), 910–920.

Dalley, M. L., & Ruscoe, J. (2003). *The abduction of children by strangers in Canada: Nature and scope*. Ottawa: Royal Canadian Mounted Police.

Efflin, J. (2019). *Death rate for suicide in the U.S. 1950–2017, by gender*. Hamburg: Statistica.

Fazel, S., Singh, J. P., Doll, H., & Grann, M. (2012). Use of risk assessment instruments to predict violence and antisocial behaviour in 73 samples involving 24,827 people: Systematic review and meta-analysis. *BMJ, 345*, e4692.

Firth, N., Barkham, M., & Kellett, S. (2015). The clinical effectiveness of stepped care systems for depression in working age adults: A systemic review. *Journal of Affective Disorders, 170*, 119–130.

Greenberg, G. (2010). *Manufacturing depression: The secret history of a modern disease*. London: Bloombury.

Hari, J. (2018). *Lost connections: Uncovering the real causes of depression—And the unexpected solutions*. New York: Bloomsbury.

Hedegaard, H., Curtin, S. C., & Warner, M. (2018). *Suicide mortality in the United States, 1999–2017*. Atlanta: CDC National Center for Health Statistics.
Joint Economic Committee. (2019). *Long-term trends in deaths of despair*. Washington: United States Senate.
Lipson, S. K., Lattie, E. G., & Eisenberg, D. (2018). Increased rates of mental health service utilization by U.S. college students: 10-year population-level trends (2007–2017). *Psychiatric Services, 70*(1), 60–63.
NICE. (2011). *Commissioning stepped care for people with common mental health disorders*. London: National Health Service. Retrieved January 21, 2019, from http://www.swscn.org.uk/wp/wp-content/uploads/2015/03/non-guidance-commissioning-stepped-care-for-people-with-common-mental-health-disorders-pdf.pdf
Our World in Data. (2019). *Global deaths in conflicts since 1400*. Retrieved from Our World in Data: https://ourworldindata.org/war-and-peace
Rhydderch, D., Krooupa, D., Goulden, R., Williams, P., Thomicroft, A., Rose, D., … Henderson, C. (2016). Changes in newspaper coverage of mental illness from 2008 to 2014 in England. *Acta Psychiatrica Scandinavia, 134*, 45–52.
Rubak, S., Sandbaek, A., Laurtzen, T., & Christensen, B. (2005). Motivational Interviewing: A systematic Review. *British Journal of General Practice, 55*(513), 305–312.
Scott, J., & Henry, C. (2017). Clinical staging models: From general medicine to mental disorders. *BJPsych Advances, 23*(5), 292–299.
Soanes, C., & Stevenson, A. (2008). *Concise Oxford English Dictionary* (11th ed.). Oxford, UK: Oxford University Press.
Stanford, S., Rovinelli Heller, N., & Warner, J. (2017). *Beyond the risk paradigm in menal health policy and practice*. London: Palgrave.
Varshney, M., Mahapatra, A., Krishnan, V., & Sinha Deb, K. (2016). Violence and mental illness: What is the true story? *BMJ, 70*(3), 223–225.
Wampold, B. E., & Imel, Z. E. (2015). *The great psychotherapy debate: The evidence for what makes psychotherapy work*. New York: Routledge.

Chapter 2
Open Access

Contents

No One Asked Me

I was visiting one of my daughters last winter. She was completing a degree in geology at a university in Western Canada. We were travelling for a day of skiing at a mountain resort about an hour away from her home when she asked me about my work on stepped care. "What is it anyway?" she asked. I decided to emphasize the rapid access, start-simple/start-strong aspect. I said my approach to stepped care provides same day care without all the questions and assessment. We start by asking people, "What is the top of mind concern for you today that you would like to address? Then we work really hard to ensure that when that person leaves in 45 or 60 minutes, s/he walks away with something useful. They are able to say, 'that was worth my time'." Without missing a beat, my daughter said, "I wish that was there when I needed it. No one ever asked me what I wanted". The experience she described at her campus counselling centre was not SC2.0. The counsellor focused on her own questions and her idea of what the problem was. She applied a lengthy, rigid, predetermined assessment protocol. My daughter said that she was disappointed by a similar approach with private practice psychologist, "and this was at my own expense!" Neither encounter was client-centric. Neither counsellor asked what she wanted or worked to ensure the first encounter was useful. Subsequent sessions seemed driven mostly by the counsellor's curiosity, agenda and questions. My daughter felt left out.

P. Cornish, *Stepped Care 2.0: A Paradigm Shift in Mental Health*,
https://doi.org/10.1007/978-3-030-48055-4_2

2.1 The Professionalization of Everyday Life

What went wrong with my daughter's attempts to access care? Both counsellors were licensed, well-trained and highly qualified. They were practicing as they had been taught. My guess is that each started the session with an open-ended question like, "tell me what led you to come in today?" I imagine each listened actively and with empathy for a minute or two. But then they got down to business. There was the requirement to follow an intake protocol of some sort. These may have varied in length and degree of structure depending on the style of each provider. The focus for both was likely on identifying risks, symptoms and formulating a conceptualization of the problem. Their questions were probably aimed at ruling out alternative diagnostic possibilities. All of them were deficit-oriented. The goal was to turn over every stone and take notice of the unpleasant material underneath. This was, of course, was well-intentioned. It was the best way, they thought, to identify the sources of her difficulty and then neutralize them. They truly wanted to help my daughter. Unfortunately, my daughter did not find the experience to be particularly engaging or fruitful. She left frustrated.

So, as mental health professionals, and help-seekers like my daughter, how did we arrive at this disconnect? For decades we have encouraged people who struggle with anxiety or depression to seek professional help. A generation of children, including my daughter, heard that message repeatedly from teachers and guidance counsellors. Public education has focused on stigma reduction in order to encourage help-seeking. There is evidence now that stigma is decreasing (Lipson, Lattie, & Eisenberg, 2018; Quartana et al., 2014). Not surprisingly, more people are seeking help. This is undoubtedly a positive development. More than ever before, people are becoming comfortable talking about their mental health to friends, loved ones and colleagues. Social and emotional learning is being incorporated in school curricula. Workplace standards for supporting mental health have been developed, and large corporations and philanthropic organizations are investing in mental health campaigns and more sophisticated employee assistance programs. While promising, these efforts lack coordination or clear direction. And in many cases, a common message encourages consultation with experts.

Allan Francis, one of the architects of the DSM IV, now laments his work on the project and the resulting medicalization of everyday life (Frances, 2013). Tom Insel, former director of the National Institute of Mental Health also expresses regrets. He oversaw approximately $20 billion dollars in spending on neurobiological research which he now admits had no impact on mental health. He now suggests we focus more on identifying social and psychological factors that contribute to well-being (Insel, 2019).

When emotionally distressing events like a death or suicide occur in a school, administrators dispatch a team of counsellors to console the children. Similar deployment of psychological crisis response teams are common in workplace tragedies. I have assumed the role of counsellor in such situations. While in theory this strategy aims to reduce risk of trauma or—in the case of suicide, contagion—I believe this is misleading, signalling to people that they should turn more to experts than each other in times of trouble. I have noticed that employees, administrators, children, parents and teachers are not especially interested in connecting with counsellors at these moments. Counsellors, in turn, seem to feel out of place, standing or sitting awkwardly on the periphery, wondering how or whether to engage. Are we interfering in what would otherwise be a natural and healthy process of community engagement? Are we effectively disempowering people by our presence?

We learned after years of promoting critical incident debriefings following traumatic events that these actually cause greater harm than good (Bledsoe, 2003). The debriefings were based on the assumption that PTSD onset could be prevented by leading all who had endured a tragic event through intensive, professionally guided exposure exercises. While there is some evidence that peer-led debriefings can be helpful, debriefings by outsiders, even those with solid mental health training have been shown to slow recovery. Current best practices suggest conducting informational sessions that emphasize the normal, healthy reactions to crisis and outline resources that could be helpful should recovery stall or symptoms deepen (Pack, 2012). When I am asked to offer to support to organizations in time of crisis, I prefer to limit my role to that of consultant to the leaders of the organization. In other words, I aim to support and empower the designated administrators who are already known to the community to provide the right information. I help them to trust their natural instincts and to supplement them with resources that are evidence-informed.

2.2 The Real Reasons for Surging Demand

Large numbers of people, including my daughter, are now ready to work on their mental health. Our public education and anti-stigma campaigns have succeeded. But instead of supporting people to work together on building healthy communities, we tend to encourage reliance on experts. Why is this so? Offering the highest level of expert support is certainly well-intentioned, especially when we are concerned about deteriorating mental health. However well-intentioned, the risk is that we could be discouraging the development of community and resilience. I think there could be darker explanations for the knee-jerk *call-in-the-experts* reaction. Stigma. While more people are comfortable with help-seeking, there is still likely reluctance to offer support to those who are emotionally troubled. It is a circular problem. We fear doing the wrong thing, or fear that someone who is troubled could be dangerous. So, we call in the experts. And the more we call upon experts to manage crisis situations, the more we reinforce the stigma. I call this the "pass-the-hot-potato" syndrome. Mental illness, odd behaviour and distress are all perceived as warning signs of danger and not only is the potato too hot to hold, we think we are being caring and responsible citizens when we rely so heavily on those with the most training.

Compounding this problem is the temptation for politicians to conflate violence with mental illness. Despite the fact that mentally ill people are less likely than those who are not to commit acts of violence, a common conservative narrative explicitly states that mental illness is the root cause of "senseless" violence. Extreme acts of violence are rarely senseless. They usually require careful planning, attention to detail and resourcefulness. Hostility is the most common factor. And hostility is not a mental illness. Neither is anger or bad behaviour. Acts of violence are most often conducted with a clear, even razor-sharp mind. Sadly, often the same people who attribute violence to mental instability are the first to suggest punishment. As such, the mental illness/violence equivalency narrative only serves to undermine efforts to invest more in mental health. Better to just lock up dangerous/crazy people and throw away the key.

Large pharmaceutical firms have distorted our perspective on mental health. They have successfully marketed the "bio-chemical disease" model of mental illness for virtually all types of human distress and dysfunction (Kirsch, 2009; Spielmans & Parry, 2010; Whitaker, 2010). These efforts are aimed at everything from depression to social anxiety to sexual dissatisfaction. Millions of people now believe that mental well-being can be achieved with medicine. This, despite the fact that clinical trial evidence for pharmaceutical treatment is weak at best and no clear biochemical mechanisms for antidepressants have ever been identified (Moncrieff, 2009; Shorter, 2011).

The fact that help-seeking is increasing suggests that stigma might be decreasing. But the picture is not so clear. Celebrating the end of stigma is premature. While there are some signs that stigma is decreasing for youth (Lipson et al., 2018), there is some evidence that stigma might actually be increasing for the general population (Mackenzie, Erickson, Deane, & Wright, 2014). Self-reports of despair and distress are increasing as is the expectation that this can be relieved either medically or professionally. But rates of mental illness have been stable for decades (Baxter et al., 2014). People are reporting greater feelings of distress but not more mental illness. While in some cases professional help is appropriate, medicalizing normal distress is not. Seeking professional help for normal distress is potentially disempowering insofar as it weakens self-reliance. In schools, on university campuses and in workplaces, authorities who observe distress are being advised to refer people for professional assessment and care. Clearly well intentioned, this rush to professionalism coincides with a pass-the-hot-potato impulse. Risk managers, fearing violence, reinforce this process. This, in turn leads back to stigmatizing distress and mental illness. We have convinced, and sometimes frightened people into thinking that mental health is both fragile and complex. It is best left to professionals.

Adding to the problem is the limited supply of experts and mental health programming. Jurisdictions that have recruited additional mental health personnel, find that the demand immediately catches up. Why is this the case? I believe the increased comfort with help-seeking combined with the medicalization of distress is contributing to a curious demand spike. The demand is soft and price-sensitive. It is soft because when professional care is either unavailable or too expensive, those experiencing only mild or moderate distress may prefer to wait and/or recover on their own. When the supply of counsellors increases, those with mild or moderate distress come rushing back until capacity is reached again. This cycle is neither sustainable nor effective in strengthening resilience. A more viable option is to encourage natural family, peer and community-based support. While there may be a need for more professional care aimed at some currently underserved populations, new investment should be aimed at health and wellness promotion, targeting families and communities directly.

2.3 Investing Upstream

I do believe we need to invest more in mental health, but not a lot more. It is more important to use existing resources differently. We should shift towards health promotion and upstream programming. Figuring out how to reconfigure existing resources will not be easy. Some new money would be well spent on system-building with close attention to the process of change. This means applying implementation science in support of innovation. Instead of hiring more people to do the same, invest new money in changing how we organize care. While there may be a need for increased investment to fill some existing gaps in mental health (e.g., low-intensity programming including walk-in clinics and e-mental health infrastructure) we may not require the additional funds in the long run. Some additional money spent now on upstream programming will be recovered as the need for downstream programming decreases.

Upstream programming involves more than public education. It requires a variety of accessible care options aimed at preventing small issues or needs from growing into more serious ones. We have some of these now for our physical wellness. Healthy food guides prepared by our departments of health are one example. Laws and policies regulate the food industry to ensure that people know the nutritional value of the foods when grocery shopping. While parks and recreation centres are often key components of urban planning, regulations on requirements are loose. How many should we have and how should they be subsidized? Where are the policies ensuring all workspaces have windows or natural light? Why don't building codes require all properties to have greenspace and trees? Restaurants and workplaces must abide by strict safety codes and food preparation practices. And although in Canada we have a psychological standard for health and safety in workplace, there are no laws to enforce it.

2.4 Starting Simple, Starting Strong

Monte Bobele, a seasoned single session trainer and colleague of mine, admits that critics sometimes dismiss his method as a *Band-Aid* solution, implying it has no real value. But the Band-Aid, he counters, is one of the most useful and elegant medical devices ever invented. It is simple, flexible, inexpensive, portable and widely accessible. More importantly, it saves lives by stopping bleeding and preventing infection. It is, therefore, ironic that critics of one-at-time therapy use it as a metaphor for inadequacy. The fact that the brand name, Band Aid, became a generic term for this popular device heightens the irony. As with Occam's razor, the simplest solution is typically the best solution. If the patient presents with a small cut, it would be absurd to engage in an exhaustive investigation into what else might be wrong. Just put on a Band-Aid! Likewise, if a person comes to a walk-in mental health clinic and says I want help to manage stress, why not start there? Is it necessary to assess for depression, for a family history of psychosis or anxiety? Of course, if simple stress management strategies fail to work, further investigation might be called for.

We argue that a trial and error approach only makes sense if simple is the default approach. We don't need to turn over every stone at the first encounter. Instead begin on the surface. With mental health issues, sometimes the problem *is* only skin-deep. To think otherwise is discriminatory. I suspect the fact that upending every stone is our current default approach speaks to the long-standing deep distrust we have for presentations of human psychic distress. We suspect something dark or ominous. We do not trust overt presentations or explicit requests of clients. Perhaps mental health professionals of all persuasions are still more under the influence of psychoanalytic theory than we thought. Do we always need to identify the deep seated, sometimes dark impulses lurking in our unconscious? Don't get me wrong. This stuff is fascinating. I loved my training in psychodynamic therapy. But this deeper analysis should not be where we begin. I reserve it as a last resort. It can make the otherwise onerous work with some of our most challenging cases both fascinating and rewarding. But only if simple solutions fail.

Self-correction, a core feature of stepped care, is much more welcome after a minor investment of energy than a major one. Self-correction doesn't make much sense in traditional practice because we are under the illusion that with careful, exhaustive, deep up-front assessment we will get it right. If clients resist, this is because they are not ready. Readiness, in this context, is just a modern variation on defensive resistance. When treatment doesn't work, it is due to client limitation. There is never any need for self-correction with such an entrenched system of confirmatory bias. In contrast, SC2.0 begins with no assumptions and no pretense on getting anything right. Assessment is not used to support our theories or justify our treatment protocols. It is used instead to tell us in a more honest, transparent and accountable fashion when we get it right and when we get it wrong.

2.5 Capturing the Moment of Readiness

Who decides what to focus on in treatment? My daughter was not asked what she wanted to talk about, nor was she asked what kind of care she wanted. Why not? Why don't we begin with trusting the person in front of us with both questions, and then bring in our expertise when needed? If we start with the perspective of the person in front of us, chances are we will connect with something that they are interested in working on. Even if, somehow, we *do* know better, chances are the person will either disagree or not be interested in our approach in our ideas. One of the first things I was taught in graduate school is that help-seekers are not looking for advice. But is beginning treatment with an exhaustive assessment followed by a treatment plan based on diagnosis really much different from advice giving? It just comes in a fancier package. Some of my colleagues say, people want to be heard, they want to tell their stories—this requires lots of time. But, I counter, that is why we are trained to be skilled listeners. A skilled listener can pull a story from someone in a matter of minutes. Listening actively and accurately is crucial for rapid alignment. It is pleasurable to be heard. And for some this may be enough. But most people would say they want more than being heard. They want a problem solved or to function and feel better. Being listened to will usually make a person feel better. But being listened to and gaining some agency and solving a problem would likely feel even better. When we target the moment of readiness, clients will feel heard. They will think or say, "Yes that's it, that's what I want to work on". They will feel aligned. And then when we help the person to see they can make headway themselves, right now, today, they feel accomplished and capable.

We know about the importance readiness for change from years of research on addictions recovery (Krebs, Norcross, Nicholson, & Prochaska, 2018). People vary in the extent that they are ready to make *prescribed* life changes. A prescribed change is one recommended by someone else. Stages of change research suggest that only about 20% of people are ready (Norcross, Krebs, & Prochaska, 2011). But this fact is often misinterpreted. Everyone is 100% ready to change something; it just might not be what others think they should change. There is usually a fair amount of disagreement on what to change. Expert driven care often prescribes a very specific change. When a therapist recommends CBT, up to 80% of people will not bite. It is not because CBT is ineffective, nor is it that people are resistant. It is more a matter of preference. Our most valued expertise is process related. But we often act like technicians. Delivering a course of CBT, without attention to process, would simply be a technical act. Identifying the issue and strategy most aligned with readiness is a process skill. Nothing is prescribed in this process. The process cannot be manualized. When someone has made the effort to reach out, and we make ourselves available right at that moment, it does not matter what we think they should do. It matters so much more what the person in front of us is ready to do.

A colleague of mine is the founder of a very successful peer support network. She, as do all who work in the organization, identifies as someone with lived experience of mental illness. She is in recovery. Her symptoms and illness come and go. Her functioning moves up and down. She, like my daughter, urges providers to be more trusting of clients' experiences and preferences. She makes impassioned pleas to mental health professionals like me to "always start with ATP!" *Ask-the-person* in front of you instead of relying on lengthy intake or screening protocols. Just ask "what is top of mind for you right now" or "what would you like to be different in your life". My colleague reminds me not to be surprised if people with lived experience have some brilliant answers.

A more efficient mental health system would be tailored to capturing the moment of readiness (Hoyt & Talmon, 2014). Our assessment and techniques would focus more on identifying the problem that is most relevant to the person and identifying the thing they are most motivated to try in an effort to resolve the problem. The approach I described to my daughter while driving to the ski hill is such a method. It is in line with single session, or one-at-a-time therapy, the drop-in counselling approach introduced and developed by Moshe Talmon in the early 1990s (Talmon, 1990). Talmon is the first to admit that "single session" is a misnomer and that he prefers to call it "therapy-one-at-a-time". But his publisher insisted on "single session" convinced it would sell more books. Monte Bobele has told me that he prefers the term "open access therapy". All three terms mean that every session is self-contained, includes a simple, very brief assessment, an intervention and some evaluation on whether the intervention was helpful. The session is meant to stand on its own, much the way a visit to your family physician is meant to achieve an outcome without any expectation of a follow-up. Of course, a follow-up is possible. Physicians often say, if you are not feeling better in 3 or 4 days, make an appointment to see me and we consider other options. An additional session is possible; it just isn't the default. As Talmon and colleagues suggest, each session is treated as if it may be the last. This fits well with the fact that the modal visit in psychotherapy is one, regardless of therapeutic approach. In other words, many people only come once no matter what, so it is important to ensure that the first encounter includes a targeted intervention.

In contrast, traditional "intake" sessions are never treated like they might be the last session. Indeed, the opposite is true. The word "intake" itself implies this is just the beginning. The whole purpose of the session is to convince the client that being *taken* into our system is a good idea. Often, like my daughter's experience, the "taking in" is all that happens. Lots of questions are asked and no intervention is offered.

2.6 Open Access

Imagine the impact on our collective health if people were to have open access to appropriate care when and where they want it. The good news is that we already have the capability. Single session (or therapy one-at-a-time) clinics are opening across Canada and increasingly other parts of the world. In Newfoundland and Labrador, help-seekers can choose between three modalities of rapid access care: web, phone, in-person. Monte Bobele suggests the term "open access care" to encompass the expansion of therapy one-at-a-time through multiple modalities. Open access in Newfoundland Labrador includes same day care through three modalities (see Fig. 2.1). With all three options, care begins immediately with minimal assessment.

1. The *Bridge the gApp* web portal: a directory listing all care options for the Province and links to a suite of e-mental health tools of varying intensity designed

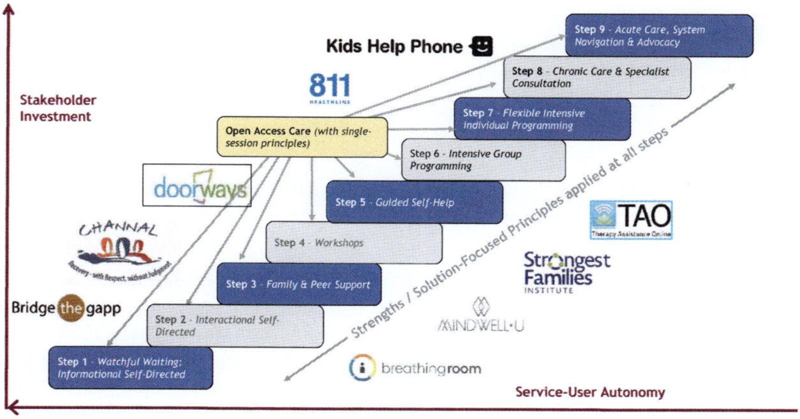

Fig. 2.1 Innovative programs accessible through the *bridge the gApp* portal in Newfoundland and Labrador

to accommodate different preferences and learning styles (i.e. *Mood Met*er self-assessment tool that points to appropriate resources; *Wall of Hope* peer forum, *Breathing Room* positive psychology self-managed depression program; *TAO*—mid-intensity blended therapist assisted self-managed treatments for depression, anxiety, relationships and substance use; *Strongest Families* telephone-led professional anxiety treatment for children and youth; *Mindwell U* 30-day mindfulness training program).

2. Three phone lines: The Provincial *811 help line* staffed by mental health professionals; The *Warmline*: Staffed by paid, highly trained peers with lived experience of mental illness; *The Crisis Text Line.*
3. *Doorways* one-at-a-time drop in clinics at 60 sites across the Province offers sessions at physical clinic spaces.

We start strong, capturing the energy that motivated the help-seeking and drawing on the existing client strengths to address the top-of-mind issues. In all three modalities, the client is introduced to the idea of trying something simple with reassurance that additional options are available should the simple approach be insufficient. This suggestion sets the foundation for a "fail-forward" approach aimed at promoting resiliency.

On the one hand, the open-access, start-strong/start-simple approach is hypnotic. It leverages hope, through the power of suggestion, that simple can be impactful. The solution-focused interview style is rooted in Ericksonian Hypnotherapy. Hope is prescribed, and beliefs instilled in the potential of untapped internal capacities. Clients draw on existing strengths and past successes to make many small differences that collectively have meaningful impact. Chaos theory, often exemplified by the butterfly effect, suggests that small events matter but predicting their effect is near impossible. Economists know this, as do successful business operators. For most businesses, continual small tweaks are the most effective way to produce sustained growth. These iterations keep clients interested and engaged. If these minor alterations fail, the impact can be moderated through vigilant monitoring and nimble adjustments. But if they succeed and compound, the rewards can be spectacular. Critics of single session therapy are correct to question whether a simple change will lead with any certainty to a specific health outcome, but chances are that with the multiple, iterative one-at-a-time micro-solutions available through an open access system, collective impact will be positive.

2.7 Failing Forward

Our SC2.0 approach suggests that failure is also okay. But this is only true if there is a wide range of treatment options. Availability of all the options is made clear at the outset for two reasons:

1. Choice from the buffet is empowering and supports ownership and buy-in.
2. Clients get a sense that, should their first choice fail, other viable options exist.

The intent of our approach is to stimulate hope and optimism while also preparing people for persistence and flexibility when results are not optimal. With full transparency, we share the full menu with clients on a first encounter (in-person, phone or on the web). One version of the menu is illustrated in the two-dimensional graphic above. For phone and in-person sessions, clients are informed that they are at the open-access point (see box in the middle of the graph), and that the open-access encounter is meant to be productive and targeted. We recommend that only experienced therapists lead these sessions. Conducting a brief focused assessment, as well as a successful intervention in a single encounter, requires both a generalist's breadth of knowledge and solid solution-focused interviewing skills. Open access sessions also demand quick, on-your-feet thinking, as well as confidence with experimenting. Therapists must be able to hone in on opportunities for capturing the moment of readiness. This is why the open-access sessions are at the mid-level of the graphic. While the open access sessions do not require the most specialized (and expensive) care, the work demands a high level of therapeutic energy.

Open access means that people can get care rapidly and through a variety of modalities. Having multiple modalities such as an online portal, telephone and text options and in-person drop-in, reduces barriers, opening up access. In line with one-at-a-time therapy principles, each open access encounter is treated as if it could be the last. This means that the encounter begins with a focused, very brief assessment. Typically, it involves a question like this: "What concern or issue is top-of-mind for you today?" While there is no proscription on the number of issues brought forward, a skilled interviewer brings focus to the issue that is most relevant at the present moment. The assumption is that motivation for working towards change will be highest for the issue that is top-of-mind. It allows the interviewer to capture the moment of opportunity for creating a solution that is of greatest relevance.

Suppose a client responds by saying "I'm feeling shock, anxiety and extreme loneliness because my partner of six years broke up with me and I really didn't see it coming". After some active listening, and a brief screening for potential suicidal risk, the interviewer might say, "Tell me what things you have done to cope so far". By identifying even the smallest of successes with coping so far, the therapist is attempting to identify existing strengths. The interviewer might also ask the client to imagine the end of the session and to picture feeling better and having the thought, "I'm glad I came. This was worthwhile." Then after a pause, the therapist could ask, "What is different as you imagine this? What has changed for you? Or what will you be doing next as a result of the session today?" These questions, posed at the outset, are deliberately hypnotic; they invite a small measure of hopefulness. They also set up realistic goal setting. In this case, the client might answer, "I would be feeling less anxious and maybe I would have a plan to help me become more active so that I don't wallow in my grief".

2.8 Informed Consent

The one-at-a-time approach is relatively new. Even newer is our SC2.0 system model. Expectancy is a key driver of mental health outcomes. If the treatment matches expectations, recovery is more likely. This presents us with both a challenge and an opportunity. Shifting expectations of stakeholders require careful and deliberate communication. But it also affords an opportunity to leverage the impact of mental health promotion. We take two approaches to meet this challenge—public education and informed consent at point of contact. Messaging the model happens on clinic websites, tear-off sheets and wellness plan/prescription pads in primary care clinics. For the broader population, the model is promoted through mental health literacy campaigns and program descriptions in online service directories.

At first point of contact, clients receive a description of SC2.0 which includes references to the one-at-a-time approach as well as the fail-forward trial and error method. SC2.0 is transparent. The provider is explicit about starting strong and simple, "I really want you to feel by the end of our meeting that this was worthwhile. To make sure this happens I will work really hard to ensure that we focus on the issue that is top-of-mind for you and better yet, that we identify some ways to began resolving it quickly. I will help you to identify strengths, capacities, and resources that you already have, but may have lost sight of. I will also share any ideas I have about resources that I think you may find helpful. Then by the end of our meeting you will already have begun building a solution. How does that sound?" This is informed consent for SC2.0.

This care-at-point of need occurs either in-person, over the phone or through chat/text interface. This start-simple/start-strong mind-set shapes the interview styles of crisis and intake workers. It is woven into the practices of therapists from all theoretical orientations – cognitive behavioural, interpersonal/dynamic and humanistic therapy. While the approach is rooted in principles of solution-focused and narrative therapy, the start-simple/start-strong attitude can be applied when disputing thought patterns, exploring relationship dynamics or developing self-worth.

Upfront assessment is minimal in open-access approaches. In some cases, it begins with only the single top-of-mind question described above. In other cases, clients may complete an open-ended single sheet with seven or eight questions in the waiting room (see Fig. 2.2). These questions can be asked over the phone, or when first joining a chat session. In some settings, a brief computerized monitoring assessment may be offered in the waiting room.

WALK-IN THERAPY CLINIC – CLIENT QUESTIONNAIRE

Date:

Name: Age: Date of birth:

Address: Phone #

1. What concern(s) have brought you here today?
2. IF 10 is the best and 1 is the worst, how are things in your life today?
   Worst 1 2 3 4 5 6 7 8 9 10 Best
3. What would be the best thing that could happen in this meeting today?
4. What is the one problem that seems most important to work on now?
5. What is it like when this problem is around?
6. Are you currently at any risk of harm to yourself or others? Yes ___ No ___
7. Remember a problem that happened any time in your life that you resolved in such a way that left you feeling proud of yourself. What did you do that you felt proud of?
8. What would someone else come to admire and respect most about you if they had months or years to get to know you? It's OK to guess.
   OR
   What would someone else like and respect most about you if they had a lot of time to get to know you?

Fig. 2.2 Single session or therapy one-at-a-time drop-in waiting room survey

2.9 Early Alignment

The success of open-access programs, as with any treatment, depends on process factors that contribute to the client experience. This is why care and connection are so much more important than cool, detached information gathering or assessment. Warmth, kindness and the promise of some immediate relief must be conveyed immediately. Alignment is primary. Information is secondary. This is true for all access modalities, including self-managed programming delivered online.

Brief, targeted screens are available for online mental health platforms. For example, the same start-simple/start-strong approach guides the organization of self-help resources offered through a web-portal. Narrative approaches guide journaling activities aimed at goal setting. With goals established, simple AI algorithms guide self-managed treatment decisions. Users are encouraged to consider a wide variety of available self-help options and to begin with one that has intuitive appeal. Instead of prescribing options based on symptom profiles, our approach is driven first by user preference, and then with return visits, through progress tracking feedback. Guidance emphasizes the importance of both preference and experimentation. Users are encouraged to balance a trial and error attitude with persistence. The AI prompts are designed to motivate and engage users. Sometimes this includes emphasizing the values of recovery that are so important to users—coping, growth, resilience, social functioning, independence and empowerment. A clinical trial indicated that the chat-based *Woebot* treatment for mood disorders was effective. Most intriguing, however, was the conclusion that the benefit came not from the cognitive-behavioural techniques taught be the chatbot, but from the relationship users developed with the cute, funny bot itself (Fitzpatrick, Darcy, & Vierhile, 2017). Just as psychotherapy with humans is only as successful as the alignment or bond with the therapist, online platforms will only be as successful as they are enticing or engaging.

2.10 No Wrong Door

In 2018, SC2.0, including open-access care was launched across the Province of Newfoundland and Labrador. Early usage and satisfaction data indicate that the program was well-received. Wait times were reduced by 65%, with some communities reporting no waiting. We collected both quantitative and qualitative satisfaction data during the initial pilot phase from a small, non-representative convenience sample. As indicated in Fig. 2.3, most people still accessed standard Step 7 individual counseling programming. However, more than half accessed low-intensity programming. Of the low-intensity programming, the drop-in Doorways clinics were most popular. Although the response rate was low and not representative of the population, close to 80% of people surveyed said that the self-managed online mental health programs available through the Bridge the gApp portal met at least some of their needs.

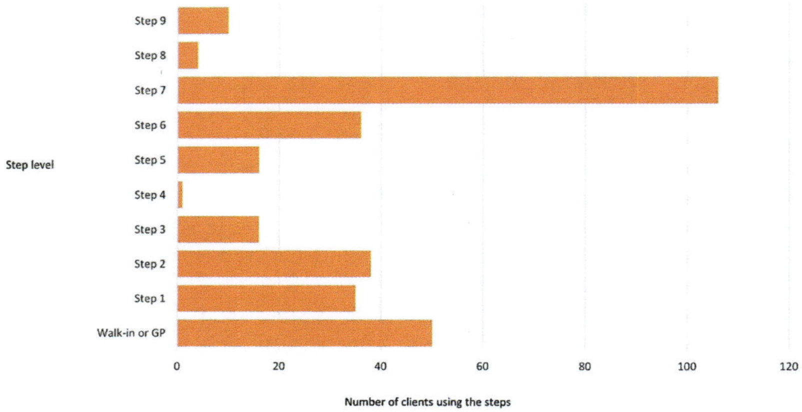

Fig. 2.3 Selected results from the Stepped Care 2.0 e-MH demonstration project (MHHC, 2019)

With open-access care, there is no wrong door. Some have argued for a single point of access to care. Integrated primary care clinics strive for this and they are an improvement over disorganized, decentralized services demarcated by professional discipline and disparate funding models. A single point of access is a good idea. It erases the contrived dichotomy between physical and mental health. A help-seeker can decide at the merged site whether to see a medical or non-medical professional. Or perhaps a more holistic option such as enrolling in a wellness program, would involve both medical and non-medical care.

As described in Chap. 6, collaborative care is central to SC2.0. However, proponents of integrated care recognize that there are some disadvantages to co-location. Not everyone will be comfortable with the one doorway. I recall students at our newly merged Student Wellness and Counselling Centre lamenting the peaceful, old counselling waiting room. While the new space, with large windows facing a forested hillside, was modern and efficient, it was noisier and busier. Some felt too exposed. Self-conscious students, anxiously awaiting their first mental health contact, had to share space with young parents and crying babies.

Open-access care introduces multiple doorways, where any door could be the right door. Through an open-access system, clients can choose between more public and private locations. For some, web access to health and mental health resources is preferred because no one would know. And the bright, noisy waiting room could be avoided. For others, human contact is essential. And still others might prefer the anonymity of a crowd, "I am just waiting here, like everyone else, alongside crying babies and people seeking refills".

Desire Paths

Twenty-five years ago, when I was working as a predoctoral intern, I commuted to work by bus and then walked half-way around the central campus bowl path to get to my office. There were signs along the path prohibiting pedestrians from walking on the grass. Judging by the criss-crossing paths, these signs were largely ignored. It made sense to me that people ignored the signs, seeking the most direct route from one building to another, or in my case from the bus stop to the Student Services Building. One day, to my surprise, a temporary fence surrounded the bowl. Construction signs replaced the keep off the grass signs. I learned that the administration had allocated funding for a 5-foot rot-iron fence to ensure the grass remained green. I have long had a layperson's curiosity about architectural design. I recalled reading something about "desire pathways"—a term for delaying construction of footpaths until the natural chosen paths were observed. I wondered to myself at the time, why the administration chose to install a rot-iron fence instead of simply paving over the routes already claimed by the community.

References

Baxter, A., Scott, K. M., Ferrari, A. J., Norman, R. E., Vos, T., & Whiteford, H. A. (2014). Challenging the myth of n "epidemic" of common mental disorders: Trends in the Global prevalence of anxiety and depression Between 1990 and 2010. *Depression and Anxiety, 31*, 506–516.

Bledsoe, B. E. (2003). Critical incident stress management (CISM): Benefit or risk for emergency services. *Prehospital Emergency Care, 7*(2), 272–279.

Frances, A. (2013). *Saving normal: An insider's revolt against out-of-control psychiatric diagnosis, DSM-5, big pharma, and the medicalization of ordinary life*. New York: Morrow.

Fitzpatrick, K. K., Darcy, A., & Vierhile, M. (2017). Delivering cognitive behavior therapy to young adults with symptoms of depression and anxiety using a fully automated conversational agent (Woebot): A randomized controlled trial. *JMIR Mental Health, 4*(2), e19.

Hoyt, M., & Talmon, M. (2014). *Capturing the moment: Single session therapy and walk-in services*. Bethel, CT: Crown House Publishing.

Insel, T. (2019). *Can smartphones solve the mental health crisis*. In *8th annual E-mental health conference: New generations new services*, BC: Vancouver.

Kirsch, I. (2009). *The emperor's new drugs: Exlpoding the antidepressant myth*. London: Bodley Head.

Krebs, P., Norcross, J. C., Nicholson, J. M., & Prochaska, J. O. (2018). Stages of change and psychotherapy outcomes: A review and meta-analysis. *Journal of Clinical Psychology, 74*(11), 1964–1979.

Lipson, S. K., Lattie, E. G., & Eisenberg, D. (2018). Increased rates of mental health service utilization by U.S. college students: 10-year population-level trends (2007–2017). *Psychiatric Services, 70*(1), 60–63.

Mackenzie, C. S., Erickson, J., Deane, F. P., & Wright, M. (2014). Changes in attitudes toward seeking mental health services: A 40-year cross-temporal meta-analysis. *Clinical Psychology Review, 34*, 99–106.

MHHC. (2019). *Newfoundland and Labrador stepped care 2.0 E-mental herālth demonstration project final report*. Ottawa: MHCC. Retrieved September 20, 2019, from https://www.mentalhealthcommission.ca/sites/default/files/2019-09/emental_health_report_eng_0.pdf

Moncrieff, J. (2009). *The myth of the chemical cure: A critique of psychiatric treatment*. London: Palgrave.

Norcross, J. C., Krebs, P. M., & Prochaska, J. O. (2011). Stages of change. *Journal of Clinical Psychology, 67*(2), 143–154.

Pack, M. J. (2012). Critical incident stress management: A review of the literature with implications for social work. *International Social Work, 56*(5), 608–627.

Quartana, P. J., Wilk, J. E., Thomas, J. E., Bray, R. M., Rae Omsted, K. L., Brown, J. M., … Hoge, C. W. (2014). Trends in mental health services utilization and stigma in US soldiers from 2002 to 2011. *American Journal of Public Health, 104*, 1671–1679.

Shorter, E. (2011). *How everyone became depressed: The rise and fall of the nervous breakdown*. New York: Oxford University Press.

Spielmans, G. I., & Parry, P. I. (2010). From evidence-based medicine to marketing-based medicine: Evidence from internal industry documents. *Journal of Bioethical Inquiry, 7*, 13–29.

Talmon, M. (1990). *Single session therapy: Maximizing the effect of the first (and often the only) therapeutic encounter*. San Francisco: Jossey Bass.

Whitaker, R. (2010). *Anatomy of an epidemic: Magic bullets, psychiatric drugs, and the astonishing rise of mental illness in America*. New York: Random House.

Chapter 3
Recovery Values and Principles

Contents

The Risk-Free (and Fun-Free) Residence

I had worked late one Thursday night. After a relaxing commute back home on my bicycle (mostly downhill), I received a text. There was an emergency in one of the residence buildings. Could I come to campus to advise? I hopped back on my bike and tackled the steep climb for the second time that day. There had been another student death by suicide. It was on the same floor of the same residence, during the same week in March as the one last year. The students, of course, were in shock. The residence student-staff were in particularly bad shape. Several months later, after some planning with the University administration, we held a half-day training for all the residence student–staff members. At the time, we thought it wise to move beyond suicide risk assessment and referral to focusing more on care and support. We hoped that by introducing them to some of the informal, positive psychology elements of the stepped care model, they could be relieved from the burden of risk management. As is often the case when I introduce people to SC2.0, I received several challenging questions at the workshop. Nothing out of the ordinary. But then during the break, one of the resident assistants approach me and said, "They are purposefully targeting you". "Who is?" I asked. "There are six students, at tables throughout the room, who knew you were coming to talk about stepped care and came with a plan to disrupt". "Why?" I asked. "Because they are angry. They don't like the model. They say it is just a way for the Counselling Centre to offload even more work on us that we are not qualified to do". Initially, I thought, they just don't understand the model. I can explain it and then they will get on board. Wrong. There

P. Cornish, *Stepped Care 2.0: A Paradigm Shift in Mental Health*,
https://doi.org/10.1007/978-3-030-48055-4_3

was an important message from students that we needed to heed. They had been traumatized by the burden of preventing the next suicide. And it was our fault. Experts can't even prevent suicide. We had inadvertently saddled students with an impossible task.

3.1 People with Lived Experience

There is no such thing as resistance in psychotherapy; it is only communication. This was the sentiment in the late Steve de Shazer's article "The Death of Resistance". Ironically, it was rejected 17 times before being published in 1984 (De Shazer, 1984). We should consider resistance to be a form of cooperation he argued. The students in residence, who were opposed to my method, and what the University had been doing for years, were communicating something very important. Recognizing this, we could begin to cooperate. They were telling us to stop what we were doing. We had gotten it all wrong. We had been burdening these young adults with impossible tasks. Even experts struggle to prevent suicides. There is, in fact, no evidence that even the most carefully developed suicide prevention or screening programs delivered by experts prevent any suicide fatalities (Harrod et al., 2014; Zalsman et al., 2016). The student leaders were right to be angry with us. They felt cheated, burnt out and traumatized. A remedy would not be found in more training. A more systemic shift was needed.

People with lived experience are central to recovery principles and mental health strategy. Their voices must be represented in all mental healthcare research, design and treatment. We needed their strong, angry messages to help us get SC2.0 right. System transformation efforts must embrace disruption. Practicing disruption itself can foster recovery. Meaningful recovery comes through empowerment. It can't happen without some agency or autonomy. Quite often this involves learning assertiveness. It might involve wresting control from others. That is what the students did at my workshop. They spoke truth to power. They disrupted me and my message. And I am thankful for this. It tripped me up so that I could fail forward with another iteration of SC2.0.

SC2.0 requires constant co-design with the most crucial stakeholders—people with lived experience and their peers. Residence leaders are, by definition, peer supporters. They are expected to lead by example and serve as mentors to fellow students. The leaders serve as the voices of their peers. The voices I heard were essential to any efforts at reforming the care ecosystem at the University.

With SC2.0, care practices evolve at both micro and macro levels. Micro-level adjustments happen as soon as students access care, when their preferences are honoured and treatment decisions are informed by outcome tracking. Micro-level care adjustment is discussed in detail in Chap. 5. Macro-adjustments occur when we welcome and attend to the kind of socio-political feedback expressed by the residence leaders attending my workshop. This macro-level monitoring includes both direct and indirect processes. Acknowledging the student protest is an example of direct monitoring. The residence leaders were participating as a captive audience in a formal setting. Their feedback was direct. Indirect socio-political monitoring is equally important. It means that those of us involved in health system transformation must be attuned to social media chatter and prepared to engage constructively. All criticism of the care ecosystem, including the new recovery-oriented programs we introduce, is grist for the mill. Protest affords an opportunity to invite those with passion to join us at the design table.

Translation or transformation of protest, anger, criticism or defensiveness into productive growth opportunities and processes are central roles for any skilled psychotherapist. As a psychodynamic therapist, I was taught to think of this as repairing therapeutic ruptures. I learned that it could be one of the most transformative elements in a course of psychotherapy. This openness to processing therapeutic failures is an example of micro-level recovery-oriented practice. With SC2.0, we extend such reflexive processing to a system level by welcoming complaints as opportunities for collaborative efforts in making structural adjustments. For example, in the case of the residence protest, student leaders were invited to re-evaluate the suicide prevention and postvention strategies. At these meetings, we considered options for moving beyond the risk-oriented policies that had eroded natural, hopeful, playful dynamics essential to a vibrant and healthy campus community. We acknowledged that efforts to professionalize resident assistant roles with training in risk assessment, gatekeeping or mental health coaching had backfired. We decided collectively that the primary responsibility of student leaders was to create conditions for a socially engaged, intellectually stimulating community. We didn't need a counsellor or an e-mental health program for that. The protesters were right—counselling is a counsellor's job, not theirs.

This reflexive analysis led us to ramp up plans to launch our embedded counsellor program. Newly hired wellness navigators had been trained in single session, one-at-a-time, walk-in counselling. The plan was to open walk-in clinics at various sites around campus. We decided to fast-track this in residence. Other sites under consideration included the International Student Advising Office and a nearby satellite campus.

Our administrative group, comprised of the directors of residences, student life and the student wellness and counselling centre spent some time reflecting on institutional policies that had taken us down the risk paradigm rabbit hole. Two of us had been there long enough to recall a decade-old consultant's report that labelled the culture in residence at the time as a "powder keg" of institutional liability. The binge-drinking culture and fraternity-like tradition of inter-house competition and identities were recognized as both sexist and unwelcoming of diversity. None of us disagreed. The organizational structures supporting this cultural tradition were problematic and needed transformation. Unfortunately, as is often the case, more attention was paid to dismantling the old structure than creating anything to replace it. Some efforts were made to develop academically engaging "living learning communities" and while these showed some promise, something was missing. I asked one of the leaders who had protested at the workshop for ideas. He said we need more support and investment in fun. I paused in thought and asked, "You know that multipurpose room, the one that we opened up all night after each of the suicides? How is that used most of the time?" He replied, "It isn't used at all". "Hmm," I said, "Why isn't it a games room? Do you have a games room?" "No," he said. "We have nothing like that".

3.2 Disease Model

So, what does the residence story have to do with recovery principles? Recovery goes beyond a disease model. In the risk-oriented residence environment, a disease model, rather than a recovery model, had been applied to detect "illness" and send it off for cure. Residence leaders had been trained to look for signs of mental deterioration and urge, even mandate those showing some "signs" to treatment. Obviously, this failed. Why did it fail? For one, it created a tense, overly serious atmosphere that infected all with fear. Who will be the next person at risk? When might the next suicide occur? This tension meant that leaders were walking on eggshells. That tension signalled that the environment was no longer safe, relaxing or inviting for open discourse, disclosure of struggle or simply playfulness.

A recovery philosophy, in contrast, assumes that anyone, whether ill or not, has internal strengths and capacities to recover, to improve functioning with or without professional treatment. It assumes that in most cases there is no malignant tumour and no need for surgery. Instead simple kindness, community and support are essential. More invasive treatment is reserved for cases that do not respond to the basic care. With the student leaders on suicide watch and the anxiety that permeated the residence halls leading up to the first anniversary, the essence of community was lost. Without that community, efforts at encouraging professional help-seeking, while well-intentioned, were likely experienced as coercive. Residence leaders had been asked to report even the mildest signs of suicidal ideation or intent to senior staff. Senior staff were expected to approach those exhibiting these signs with an air of concern that was also ripe with tension. In the absence of a safe, relaxing atmosphere, perhaps those at risk of suicide retreated into isolation for fear of being mandated to treatment.

3.3 The Recovery Movement

According to the US-based Substance Abuse and Mental Health Services Administration (SAMHSA), mental health recovery is "a process of change through which individuals improve their health and wellness, live a self-directed life, and strive to reach their full potential" (SAMHSA, 2020). The Mental Health Commission of Canada (MHCC) states that "the concept of 'recovery' in mental health refers to living a satisfying, hopeful, and contributing life, even when a person may be experiencing ongoing symptoms of a mental health problem or illness.

Recovery journeys build on individual, family, cultural, and community strengths and can be supported by many types of services, supports, and treatments" (MHCC, 2020).

Recovery is not a new concept. It has been fundamental to work on addictions for over a century. It is practiced to this day in 12-step groups. As with addictions, recovery principles were a product of long-fought battles waged by people with lived experience of mental illness. These were battles of resistance to power. The late French philosopher Michel Foucault might warn us now that meaningful recovery for some of our most marginalized is a false promise because powerful institutions cannot be easily challenged. He asks "Is it surprising that prisons resemble factories, schools, barracks, hospitals, which all resemble prisons?" (Foucault, 1995, p. 228). The hope lies, however, in the fact of "where there is power, there is resistance" (Foucault, 1978). The modern conceptualization of madness as an illness, according to Foucault, is no better than medieval depictions of possession by evil spirits. Illness and cure may even be worse, cloaked as they are in the guise of scientific neutrality. In this context, the possibility of recovery—being able to function despite distress and symptoms—is the possibility of freedom and autonomy.

The recovery movement can be traced back the establishment of the *Alleged Lunatic's Friend Society* in England in 1845 and the Anti-Insane Asylum Society in Illinois at the time of the Civil War (Frese & Davis, 1997). The movement expanded in 1907 when Clifford Beers created the National Committee for Mental Hygiene, later to become the National Mental Health Association and known today as Mental Health America. Beers collaborated with Clarence Hincks in Canada to establish the Canadian National Committee for Mental Hygiene known today as the Canadian Mental Health Association. Both groups continue to challenge the medical establishment to adopt more collaborative models of care and most recently are working to elevate and legitimize the role of peer-led mental services offered by trained people with lived experience. The UK-based Royal College of Psychiatrists published an editorial in 2010 stating the evidence supports recovery principles. They endorsed the recovery model as "a social movement that is influencing mental health service development around the world" (Warner, 2010). Recovery is now becoming so mainstream that it may no longer classify as a social movement.

3.4 Recovery Values, Principles and Assumptions

UK psychologist, Mike Slade defines recovery as comprising "full symptom remission, full or part-time work or education, independent living without supervision by informal carers, and having friends with whom activities can be shared, all sustained for a period of two years" (Slade & Longden, 2015).

A recovery model assumes that psychological and psychiatric problems either cannot or need not be cured. It is impossible to cure something that cannot be proven to exist. How can you cure a mental illness or just plain bad behaviour when we can't clearly identify the mechanism that needs curing? There is not a shred of evidence for biological mechanisms associated with mental illness (Moncrieff, 2009). Likewise, we have no inkling of an internal mechanism that might underlie deviant or anti-social behaviour. How would we know if we have cured something if we don't know what we are curing? An infected wound is cured with evidence that the skin has healed. I think of Foucault again: "People know what they do; frequently they know why they do what they do; but what they don't know is *what* what they do does" (Foucault, 1988). If we don't know what the *what* is that we are trying to cure, maybe we should stop trying.

A care system based on the concept of recovery is independent of risk, personal and structural deficits, and illness. By this I mean that recovery models assume that wellness programming benefits those who are not ill or not engaging in problematic behaviors just as much as they can help those in trouble. It provides health and wellness for all. It is upstream. It is not reactionary. The opening story in this chapter illustrates how care delivered in the context of our current risk paradigm only prepares a community to react after it is too late. The best prevention strategy comes not from risk detection or risk prohibition (e.g. amputating the campus drinking culture) but through community development.

According to the Mental Health Commission of Canada, "the dignity of risk or the right to failure" is important in work with people with emotional challenges or disabilities and "it refers to the importance of respecting a person's right to take risks as part of personal growth" (MHCC, 2015). Risk is essential to the development of resilience, which in turn, is a foundation for growth. There is tension and some disagreement among proponents of recovery on how to balance the right to risk and the obligation for practitioners to intervene when safety could be jeopardized (Davidson et al., 2006). However, a shift in the risk paradigm, towards a more collaborative engagement of this tension can maximize empowerment while minimizing threats to safety.

As reported in the APA Monitor, health care professionals, researchers and persons with lived experience agree on 10 core principles underlying a recovery philosophy (APA, 2012). As illustrated in Table 3.1, all 10 of these principles are applied in SC2.0. They are in fact *the* principles of SC2.0.

3.5 Recovery in Practice

As we began to implement SC2.0 across the province of Newfoundland and Labrador, we quickly discovered the power of peer support in both the treatment process and as a key driver of successful implementation. We learned that the Province's *Towards Recovery* strategy was adopted through a rare process of political non-partisanship (Government of Newfoundland and Labrador, 2017). It was advanced through the leadership of people with lived experience who sat on an all-party committee tasked with making recommendations for broad mental health system change. How did this consensus arise? Over the past two decades, persons with lived experience, including several local celebrities, found their voices heard

Table 3.1 Recovery principles and Stepped Care 2.0

Principle	Description	Application in SC2.0
Self-direction	Consumers determine their own pathway to recovery	Consumer preference, rather than simply symptom severity or diagnosis, is central to treatment decision-making
Individualized and person-centred	There are multiple pathways to recovery based on individual's unique strengths, needs, preferences, experiences and cultural backgrounds	On first contact, no assumptions are made about what will work in treatment. Instead of a lengthy assessment, the focus is on the issue that is top-of-mind for the consumer and initial solutions are informed by consumer's previous successes or coping strategies
Empowerment	Consumers can choose among options and participate in all decisions that affect them	A full range of options is outlined on first contact as well as an opportunity to consider additional options drawn from consumers' experiences
Holistic	Recovery focuses on people's entire lives, including mind, body, spirit and community	When considering options for care, the graphic representation of the model includes consideration of community resources related to mind, body and spirit
Nonlinear	Recovery isn't a step-by-step process, but one based on continual growth, occasional setbacks and learning from experience	The value of trial and error and "failing forward" is explicitly stated in first contact and throughout the care continuum
Strengths-based	Recovery builds on people's strengths	Strengths and capacities are assessed and discussed regularly through continuous, collaborative, objective therapeutic measurement
Peer support	Mutual support plays an invaluable role in recovery	The value of peer reciprocity (giving and receiving support) is emphasized at all step levels as a potentially empowering opportunity
Respect	Acceptance and appreciation by society, communities, systems of care that consumers themselves are crucial to recovery	Participation of people with lived experience in treatment, care system design and evaluation is considered a requirement for implementation of SC2.0
Responsibility	Consumers are responsible for their own self-care and journeys of recovery	Responsibility for self-care and the journey of recovery is emphasized at every care point. For example, consumers are informed that we need their assistance in getting the care right: They are encouraged to try other options or return for additional visits if upon reflection the approach taken proved unhelpful. The responsibility for trial and error, persistence and self-correction is made clear as part of the informed consent process
Hope	Recovery's central, motivating message is a better future—That people can do and do overcome obstacles	Hope, optimism and the belief in the capacities of consumers are infused throughout the care continuum which draws on principles of narrative, solution-focused and positive psychology

through a variety of local mass media channels. Persons with lived experience organized around charity events spoke on "open-line radio", a daily broadcast that just about everyone listened to, including politicians of all stripes.

With government and the people aligned on the task of massive system transformation, the Province attracted the attention of national and international organizations with missions to advance system reform. Newfoundland and Labrador became a focal point for the Mental Health Commission of Canada as well as organizations in the United Kingdom, Australia and New Zealand that been working on innovation in mental health for years. Our own development of SC2.0 was generously funded by both the Provincial and Federal governments through a series of development, demonstration and research grants. Most recently, the National office of the Canadian Mental Health Association (CMHA) has taken an interest in scaling up peer support across the country. They are particularly interested in the potential for instilling recovery values across the care continuum by implementing their *Recovery College* program within the context of SC2.0.

Recovery values can lift stigma associated with mental health and addictions. In Canada, mental health services are not funded on parity with other healthcare programs. And addictions programming is the poor cousin of mental health treatment. The disparity is worrisome as we witness a deepening opioid addiction crisis. Attempts at integration have been made to rectify the imbalance. But policies aimed at amalgamating through restructuring have been largely superficial, limited to name changes like *Community Mental Health and Addictions*. The workforce remains divided and programming disconnected despite concurrent disorder rates ranging from 20 to 80%. My colleague at McGill University, Mary Bartram, offers theoretical grounds for bridging the divide between mental health and addictions practice (Bartram, 2019, 2020). A common assumption, Bartram observes, is that addictions recovery requires abstinence, whereas mental health recovery is possible without full symptom remission. Harm reduction approaches are being embraced by some practitioners, but abstinence dominates community-based AA programs. Bartram proposes the two-continuum model advanced by Cory Keyes (Keyes, 2007) be adapted for harm reduction approaches. Just as some with serious mental illness can flourish, those with severe substance use disorders might function well and without harm. I look forward to the day when the term mental health includes addictions, and work like Bertram's, takes us a step closer.

SC2.0 is both a recovery and harm reduction model. Innovation demands risk-taking as does collaborative trial and error treatment planning. As argued in Chap. 1, SC2.0 embraces risk and, in doing so, aims to reduce harm. By sharing risk and responsibility broadly with all stakeholders, especially help seekers, harm is reduced and opportunity for recovery maximized. Providers risk trusting clients with a harm reduction approach. Providers believe in the capacities of people who are vulnerable, disoriented with symptoms, or managing a substance use disorder. We trust the person, their capacities, their readiness and their story until there might be reasons to assume otherwise. This trust increases alignment and safety.

As a long-standing advocacy organization for those with mental health and addictions, the CMHA does likewise. The CMHA is a proponent of the dual continuum model, recovery programming, peer support and stepped care. Their version of stepped care is illustrated in Fig. 3.1. Of note are the two lowest steps that target the largest segment of the population. The CMHA recognizes the value of both formal and informal community-based supports. In both cases, these programs are owned and operated by people with lived experience. Acknowledging the potential of both trained (formal) and untrained (informal) peer systems generates respect for, and empowerment of, all people with lived experience. The CMHA offers training for mental health professionals and works to equip the general public with increased capacities to support each other.

In our work with the CMHA and representatives of other peer networks and organizations, we are discovering that the distinction between steps—with or without peer support—is not as obvious as depicted in Fig. 1.2 (in Chap. 1). For example, we have learned that peers can have an important role in greeting people in clinic waiting rooms, providing information on local community resources, or they may bring value simply by sitting in a quiet nook alongside a person in distress. As indicated in Fig. 3.2, this initial contact work could involve step 1 information sharing or step 3 supportive listening. Peers can be trained to help people navigate self-help resources (at step 2). They can be trained to co-lead or lead educational workshops at step 4. They could also help oriented people to therapist-assisted eMH programming or, with proper training, provide eMH coaching under the guidance of professionals (step 5). Peers could even assist in co-facilitating intensive therapy groups (step 6). They could help clients with homework assigned in individual therapy (step 7). Likewise, peers could assist in chronic care settings. Professionals, including physicians, psychiatrists, nurses and social workers at steps 7–9 could

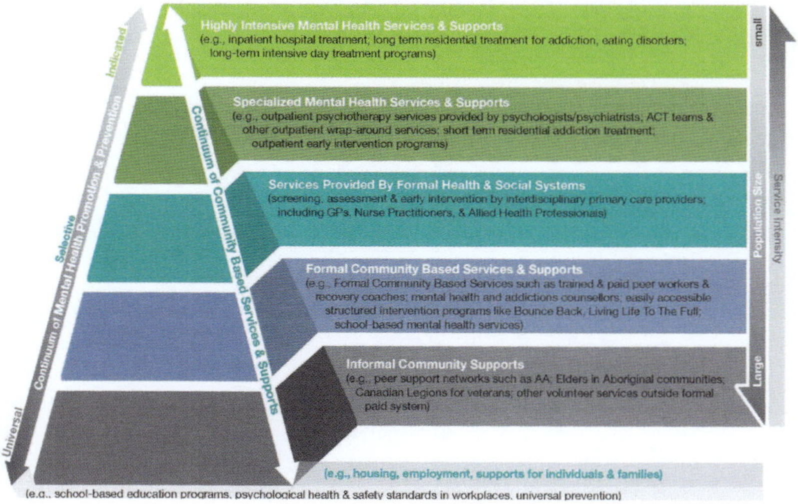

Fig. 3.1 CMHA version of stepped care (CMHA, 2018)

conduct a warm handoff to a peer that might help people get started with rehabilitation work, including exercise or navigation and transition to other points of community care. The possibilities of formal peer support in collaboration with professional programs are depicted in the lower half of Fig. 3.2. Informal peer-support activities operating independently of the formal care system are illustrated in the top part of Fig. 3.2.

Why is consumer participation so important for recovery-oriented mental health and addictions care? In this chapter, a central assumption is that co-designed care is better care. Experts have years of formal training and consumers have years of lived experience. Recovery models attempt to integrate these very different types of knowing. The chapter opened with a story of disruption and tension. The tension is productive. Without welcoming the tension, the suicide prevention strategy at Memorial University would not have advanced. Peer involvement not only facilitates care system self-correction—as was the case in the residence—it also enhances access and quality of care by reducing stigma, building trust and stimulating empowerment. One of the most promising roles for peers, described in more detail in Chap. 6, is the sense of purpose and value peers experience by giving back. This includes both giving back directly to others through care programs and indirectly by participating in care system design teams.

Many questions naturally arise as we bring together professionals and non-professionals, providers and consumers of programs. A question of boundaries is an obvious challenge. When I was in graduate school, I recall one of my professors saying, "Boundaries are crossed all the time in our work; the key is to manage these crossings appropriately". Without any boundary crossings, there will be limited connection, missed opportunities for correction, reduced creativity and no productive tension. Growth happens when we are prepared to risk and persist through failure. Rigid boundaries prohibit risk, so it is feared and avoided. Without risk, failure does not happen, resilience does not develop and growth is impossible.

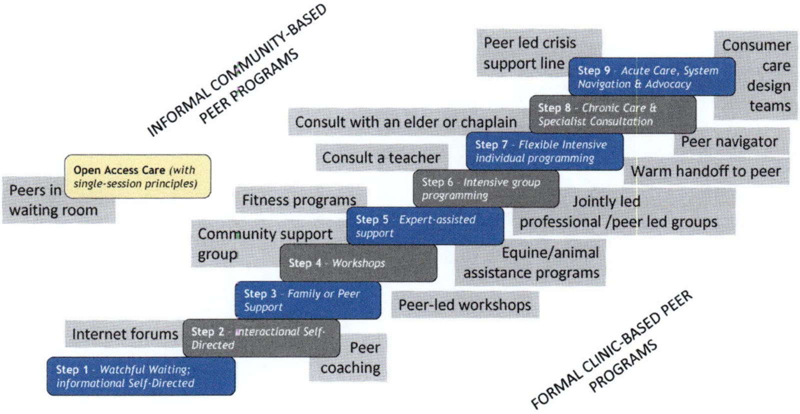

Fig. 3.2 Potential role for peers in Stepped Care 2.0

3.6 Research on Recovery

Recovery models are optimistic. One assumption is that a large portion of people with severe and persistent mental illness, including schizophrenia, can recover and function well in society. Research supports this, indicating that up to 40% of people diagnosed with schizophrenia achieve social recovery—can function socially and economically, and approximately 20% achieve full recovery—the complete absence of symptoms (Lambert et al., 2008). Another core assumption is that empowerment is a key driver for positive mental health treatment outcomes. Empowerment is a broad concept that includes psychological insight, autonomy, internal locus of control, self-efficacy, meaningful social connectedness, shared or collaborative power and vocational participation. All these factors lead to better coping with the symptoms of mental illness (Tew et al., 2012). Studies show that a combination of psychological insight, including acceptance of diagnosis, is associated with good outcomes, but only if internalized stigma is low (Caveti et al., 2012). In other words, the type of insight into the illness matters. Low internalized stigma means that illness does not define or restrict a person's self-concept. While the facts of the illness are accepted, these do not interfere with a belief in one's capacity to have a purposeful and meaningful life.

Peer support has been shown to have recovery outcomes on par with professional care (Bellamy et al., 2017). But the research also indicates an added unique benefit from peer support. Self-efficacy increases through peer support, particularly for those providing the support, more than it does for people who only receive professional care (Mahlke et al., 2017). Active involvement in clinical decision-making, a core principle of recovery, has been found to increase patient satisfaction, treatment adherence and clinical outcomes. Unfortunately, the majority of specialists tend not to encourage patient involvement especially for those with more severe illnesses.

3.7 Neoliberal Critique

While the research on recovery models is promising, some sociologists and economists question the motives (Field and Reed, 2016). Is the recovery movement simply a neo-liberal ruse to offload government responsibility for mental healthcare onto our most vulnerable citizens? Does it aim to privatise care through the illusion of choice among low-quality care options? The argument is that commodifying mental health recovery resources along a spectrum of self-help, peer led, online programs and care from least to most expensive professionals constitutes a conservative economic policy aimed at saving money and reducing public commitment to quality healthcare. In other words, recovery models can be used to support neoliberal policy aimed at reducing the size of government in favour of further corporatization of healthcare.

This is valid criticism. It would be naive to think that these forces are not at play. Healthcare spending is one of the biggest ticket items for government. There are large global players that dominate pricing of pharmaceuticals and information management. Healthcare, including mental health, is profitable. With these developments, regulation has never been more important. It is increasingly important for protecting electronic health information, the use of data and for policing pharmaceutical research and marketing. It is equally important for monitoring the development, quality and impact of new lower intensity mental health options including community-based recovery programs. There will continue to be entrepreneurial innovations in this space especially now that mental health has become a high priority for a broad range of stakeholders.

Given the growing public interest for improving mental health, governments will need to invest more, not less in healthcare budgets. However, the new investment should not be aimed at more of the same. We do not need more physicians, social workers, nurses, psychologists or psychiatrists. We need to invest in different ways of practicing, organizing and regulating existing services. This means investing in training and system infrastructure that support innovation while maintaining safety and improving outcomes. Our current care models have very low accountability through self-regulated professions that are not making use of data to maximize outcomes. If we do not change this, the only ones that will have and use the data are the large telecommunication corporations. Without government investment in system building, the neo-liberal ruse critique will prove correct.

3.8 Staging Versus Recovery

Most stepped care models involve clinical staging (Cross et al., 2014; Scott & Henry, 2017). Sometimes these are referred to as pathways models. The goal is to determine the best treatment pathway as soon as possible. Pathways are built in accordance with triage principles. Before the development of stepped care, people would be screened for symptom severity and those with the most severe symptoms get treatment sooner, whereas those with mild or moderate symptoms would have to wait. Pathways stepped care systems triage more efficiently, reducing wait times and ensuring all help-seekers, regardless of symptom severity, get care as soon as possible.

Staging and pathways stepped care models emerged approximately 20 years ago, first in the United Kingdom, then in Europe, Australia and New Zealand. At the same time that the staging model was being scaled across the United Kingdom, recovery principles were being introduced and a predictable tension emerged between the expert-driven staging approach and the more flexible patient preference-oriented practices that were being recommended.

The pathway/staging approach is premised on the assumption that assessment and diagnoses inform the choice of step level. A thorough assessment will yield a wealth of information that the clinician could interpret to recommend the correct treatment plan at the outset. Treatment decision-tree algorithms are created to signal pathways based on symptom scores. Typically, those with high symptom scores take a more direct pathway to intensive specialized care, whereas those with low or moderate symptoms will first proceed to lower steps. Stepping up or down only occurs when symptom levels change. The focus tends to be directed mostly to those actively seeking help in clinic settings. There is less attention to health promotion and illness prevention. Only treatments that have been reliably supported through independent clinical trials are considered. Close attention is paid to ensuring the fidelity of practice to the evidence-based treatment manuals.

SC2.0 is not a staging model. Nor does it determine pathways as described above. In contrast, it is a recovery model of stepped care. Unlike the staging model, it begins with minimal assessment. Instead, the help seeker's concept of the issue is taken at face value and practical, common-sense solutions are worked on immediately. This is in line with the start-simple/start-strong principle described in Chap. 2. Treatment planning is more flexible, and preference-based. Care plans are developed collaboratively. The provider outlines expectations for both parties: what the help-seeker can expect from the provider and what the provider expects from the help-seeker. Care step levels are selected to match readiness for, and interest in, meeting the expectations associated with the level of care. The assessment initially is subjective and intuitive—driven by the recovery-oriented interviewing style. The interviewer attends to signs of alignment. With the full range of step levels in mind, inquiries are made of the help-seeker's capacities, strengths and functioning level.

Evidence is conceptualized differently with recovery models. While evidence-based treatments supported by clinical trials are valued, the broader approach to data and evidence allows for the inclusion of innovative approaches that are less conducive to controlled research. Therapeutic measurement allows for some trial and error. The evidence for the treatment comes from the ongoing assessment reviewed by both the help-seeker and the provider. This collaborative review of the data is a powerful validation method. It requires a progress tracking system that is visible to both provider and help-seeker. Finally, given the openness to treatments that may not be evaluated in controlled settings, a wider range of formal and informal treatment resources are considered. Some programs may have only preliminary research support. They may also involve social prescriptions to informal community resources like AA, a yoga class or local support groups. Stepped care features of staging/pathways models are compared to those of recovery models in Table 3.2.

3.9 The Ethics of SC2.0

As we began implementing SC2.0, some colleagues questioned the model on ethical grounds. A common perception is the one-at-a-time (single session) approach oversimplifies what may be complex illnesses. Critics worry that some help seekers may feel that their serious issues are being dismissed or minimized. The trial-and-error approach is risky. If we don't get it right the first time, maybe help-seekers will become discouraged and drop out. What about people who are vulnerable? Would they be able to tolerate "fail forward"? If we are trying innovative approaches without a rock-solid evidence base, are practitioners more vulnerable to malpractice claims? Is SC2.0 ethical care, or is it a cost-saving measure that stretches resources too thin?

SC2.0 aims to improve efficiencies. This includes increasing the capacity for providers to see more people. Will this increased caseload lead to burn out and poorer care? With less up-front assessment and higher caseloads, record-keeping changes. There may be less time for record-keeping and less data obtained at the outset. Does this meet the standards or guidelines for practice of my profession? I have heard this question from social workers, psychologists and counsellors. I counter with my own question: What specifically do the guidelines say about caseloads, note-taking and quality of care? Take records for example. Most guidelines require date of treatment, name of help-seeker and some description of the problem and intervention. They do not require a specific level of detail. Records do not have to use full sentences or tell a rich story.

Ethical practice in the context of recovery values means balancing risk and opportunity with security and safety. SC2.0 introduces risk as an opportunity for growth and resilience. While ethical codes tend to focus more on risk management, it is possible to integrate recovery principles in a way that nudges gently beyond the dominant risk paradigm. I am most familiar with the Canadian Psychological Association's Code of Ethics. It is organized around four high-level principles ranked by priority. The highest level principle is *respect for the dignity persons and peoples*. SC2.0 supports this with its emphasis on client centricity, choice, empowerment, strengths and capacities. SC2.0 also supports Principle 1 with emphasis on detailed informed consent specifying expectations associated with the care model.

Table 3.2 Staging/pathways versus recovery stepped care models

Stepped care practices	Staging/pathways model	Recovery model
Regions practiced	UK, Europe, Australia, NZ	Canada, UK
Assessment	Screening and thorough assessment upfront—Purpose is to detect/address risk and conduct triage	Minimal upfront assessment, solution focus + "fail forward" initially; deep assessment only when there is "a mystery"
Treatment planning	Decision tree—Pre-determined pathways	Flexible—No pre-determined pathways
Target population	Clinic focus: Treatment priority is for active help-seekers with severe symptoms	Whole population focus: Prevention and treatment for all regardless of severity
Outcomes measured	Symptoms/deficits; treatment fidelity	Patient readiness, therapeutic alignment/engagement, functioning, capacities
Sources of evidence	Independent randomized, clinical trial results	Trial and error programming managed through continuous therapeutic measurement
Intervention settings	Medically-based formal clinic and hospital settings	Multiple sectors—Medical, community-based, educational and informal settings

The next principle is *responsible caring*. SC2.0 expands care options, eliminates wait times and enhances outcomes by up to 50% through ongoing therapeutic measurement (Miller et al., 2015). The third principle is *integrity of relationships*. Therapeutic alignment is managed transparently through continuous, objective measurement, collaborative treatment planning and explicitly stated goals, expectations and responsibilities. The fourth principle, *responsibility to society*, is enhanced through SC2.0 with expanded upstream, whole population care and interventions.

3.10 Perching and Nesting

I have often wondered how spaces could be designed to support or encourage certain types of activity, or how design can be adapted to find the right combination of security, warmth and openness. I was fortunate enough to receive an inheritance about 20 years ago that allowed me to purchase a wooded property on a rugged hillside near the ocean in Newfoundland. I had been introduced to architect, Robert Mellin, who specializes in resurrecting the vernacular *outport* fishing village architecture typical of the Fogo Island region of the Province. Robert designed a tall, long, rectangular *saltbox* house with 64 windows for my wooded hillside property. The idea was that this bright red structure would stand tall and strong against the ferocious North Atlantic gales while also melding with the surrounding landscape. It would be both protected from and transparent to nature.

Inside, the home was open, with high ceilings supported by great fir beams. The windows and skylights brought the adjacent natural landscape inside while allowing panoramic views of the cold churning ocean from every vantage point. The terra cotta tinted, heated concrete floor and massive slate clad new England fireplace brought warmth to the steely, hard surfaces that mirrored the resilient outdoor rocky landscape. While open and high, the spaces had cosy nooks. The children's rooms reached up steep peaked ceilings to a centrepiece skylights. The loft beds afforded shelter below and the hatchways at the foot of each suspended bed allowed for retreat to a cosy hidden pathway connecting the three bedrooms. All features of the home embraced a tension between the vast, wondrous, stunningly beautiful, but unrelenting forces of nature and the draw of safe, warm, protective alcoves.

Frank Lloyd Wright's work expressed this dialectic. All creatures, including humans, prize both protection, warmth and safety as well as perspective on vast open spaces. We need a room with a view. A student at the School of Architecture at Taliesin in Scottsdale, Arizona comments on the experience of living in one of Wright's student prairie desert designs: "It's a sense of freedom that I had never felt before. And it's a powerful thing", it sits on a cantilever so that it feels like "you're hanging, in this sort of nest, this perch … You're protected [from nature], but you're not separated" (Catalfamo, 2018).

This balance between hanging (or perching) and nesting is a metaphor for the vibrant, dynamic and ethically grounded SC2.0 recovery-oriented practice. There are multiple doorways for rapid, alternate routes to safety. Once safely inside, alignment and attention to care bring immediate feelings of warmth and comfort. At the same time, the visitor can view both the forest and the trees. The whole care ecosystem, both inside and out, is visible from every vantage point. There is freedom to move around, step up, down, inside and out. The entire system is transparent. It is also adaptable. As the climate and seasons fluctuate, furniture can be moved to adjust perspectives inward or out, curtains can be drawn or opened, fine-tuning the balance between exposure to the elements or recharging in the comfort of the fire, on heated floors or in cosy corners.

Meaningful healthy architectural design need not be reserved for people like me who are privileged. In British Columbia, philanthropists, mental health innovators and the Provincial Government partnered to develop integrated youth wellness hubs. Recovery principles were central to the project. Stepped care is also a key element. *Foundry BC* is the name chosen by youth to represent strength, resilience and the importance of finding a place that is home. The interior design was also driven by youth values and needs. Waiting areas are modern, vast, comfortable and colourful but also have cosy private nooks. The space is vibrant, bright and hopeful. Dynamic interior design is actually an inexpensive way to leverage recovery as well as multiple determinants of health. It is a one-time cost, and in this case funded by eager donors. Foundry brings health inspiring infrastructure and architecture to some of the least privileged and most vulnerable in our population—homeless, traumatized and/or emotionally distressed youth.

Don't Talk to Strangers

Don't talk to strangers! Who hasn't heard this warning? A recovery-oriented system would encourage more talking to strangers. I ordered a ride through Uber recently. The car arrived after about 2 minutes. As I was about to step into the back seat, the driver rolled down the front passenger window and exclaimed, "Get in the front, this is Uber not a taxi". He told me he says this to all customers and that it is almost always well-received. He described it as a gesture of kindness, one that makes a small but meaningful difference to the day of each rider. Some passengers, he continued, who might appear tense, angry or otherwise unhappy, warm up instantly with the invitation. Once when he witnessed this softening with one passenger, he asked what her plans were for the rest of the day. She sighed and said, "Well, I'm going to visit some of my girlfriends. I got divorced a few months ago, and I have been working on spending more time with them since then". I then shared with the driver that I believed more kindness among strangers is important to mental health. I added that his gesture for me to sit in the front seat that morning had boosted my mood and outlook on life. I explained that just before he arrived, I had been preoccupied with some recent bad news, but that his gesture, and our conversation, allowed me to leave the unproductive thoughts behind. Strangers, I thought with a smile on my face as I headed into the airport, are some of our best allies for mental health recovery.

References

APA. (2012). Recovery principles. *Monitor on Psychology, 43*(1), 55.

Bartram, M. (2019). Toward a shared vision for mental health and addiction recovery and well-being: An integrated two-continuum model. *Journal of Recovery in Mental Health, 2*, 2371–2376.

Bartram, M. (2020). 'It's really about wellbeing': A Canadian investigation of harm reduction as a bridge between mental health and addiction recovery. *International Journal of Mental Health and Addiction* 20–43. https://doi.org/10.1007/s11469-020-00239-7

Bellamy, C., Schmutte, T., & Davidson, L. (2017). An update on the growing evidence base for peer support. *Mental Health and Social Inclusion, 21*(3), 161–167.

Catalfamo, K. (2018, April 16). The Desert Architecture School where students build their own sleeping quarters. *Atlas Obscura*. Retrieved December 20, 2019, from https://www.atlasobscura.com/articles/taliesin-west-desert-shelters

Caveti, M., Kvrgic, S., Beck, E., Rusch, N., & Vauth, R. (2012). Self-stigma and its relationship with insight, demoralization, and clinical outcome among people with schizophrenia spectrum disorders. *Comprehensive Psychiatry, 53*(5), 468–479.

CMHA. (2018). *Mental health in the balance: Ending the health care disparity in Canada*. Toronto: CMHA. Retrieved October 18, 2019, from https://cmha.ca/wp-content/uploads/2018/09/CMHA-Parity-Paper-Full-Report-EN.pdf

Cross, P. M., Hermens, D. F., Scott, E. M., Ottavio, A., McGorry, P. D., & Hickie, I. B. (2014). A clinical staging model for early intervention youth mental health services. *Psychiatric Services, 65*(7), 939–943.

Davidson, L., O'Connell, M., Tandora, J., Styron, T., & Kangas, K. (2006). The top ten concerns about recovery encountered in mental health system transformation. *Psychiatric Services, 57*(5), 640–645.

De Shazer, S. (1984). The death of resistance. *Family Process, 23*, 11–17.

Field, B. I., & Reed, K. (2016). The rise and fall of the mental health recovery model. *The International Journal of Psychosocial Rehabilitation, 20*(2), 86–95.

Foucault, M. (1978). *The history of sexuality, Vol. 1: An introduction*. (R. Hurley, Trans.) New York: Vintage.

Foucault, M. (1988). *Madness and civilization: A history in the age of reason*. New York: Vintage.

Foucault, M. (1995). *Discipline and punish: The birth of the prison*. (A. Sheridan, Trans.) New York: Vintage.

Frese, F. J., & Davis, W. W. (1997). The consumer-survivor movement, recovery, and consumer professionals. *Professional Psychology: Research and Practice, 28*(3), 243–245.

Government of Newfoundland and Labrador. (2017). *Towards recovery: A vision for a renewed mental health and addictions system for Newfoundland and Labrador*. St. John's: Government of Newfoundland and Labrador. Retrieved December 10, 2019, from https://www.health.gov.nl.ca/health/all_party_committe_report.pdf

Harrod, C. S., Goss, C. W., & DiGuiseppi, C. (2014). Interventions for primary prevention of suicide in university and other post-secondary educational settings (Review). *Cochrane Database of Systematic Reviews*, (10), 1–88.

Keyes, C. L. (2007). Promoting and protecting mental health as flourishing. *American Psychologist, 62*(2), 95–108.

Lambert, M., Nader, D., Schacht, A., Wagner, T., Hundemer, H. P., Karow, A., … Schimmelmann, B. G. (2008). Rates and predictors of remission and recovery during 3 years in 392 never-treated patients with schizophrenia. *Acta Psychiatrica Scandinavica, 118*, 220–229.

Mahlke, C. I., Priebe, S., Heumann, K., Daubmann, A., Wegscheider, K., & Bock, T. (2017). Effectiveness of one-to-one peer support for patients with severe mental illness—A randomised controlled trial. *European Pscyhiatry, 42*, 103–110.

MHCC. (2015, January 2). *Guidelines for recovery-oriented practice: Hope, dignity, inclusion.* Retrieved from MHCC: https://www.mentalhealthcommission.ca/sites/default/files/2016-07/MHCC_Recovery_Guidelines_2016_ENG.PDF

MHCC. (2020, January 2). *What is recovery.* Retrieved from Recovery: https://www.mentalhealthcommission.ca/English/what-we-do/recovery

Miller, S. D., Hubble, M. A., Chow, D., & Seidel, J. (2015). Beyond measures and monitoring: Realizing the potential of feedback-informed treatment. *Psychotherapy, 52*(4), 449–457.

Moncrieff, J. (2009). *The myth of the chemical cure: A critique of psychiatric treatment.* London: Palgrave.

SAMHSA. (2020, January 2). *SAMHSA's working definition of recovery.* Retrieved from https://store.samhsa.gov/system/files/pep12-recdef.pdf

Scott, J., & Henry, C. (2017). Clinical staging models: From general medicine to mental disorders. *BJPsych Advances, 23*(5), 292–299.

Slade, M., & Longden, E. (2015). Empirical evidence about recovery and mental health. *BMC Psychiatry, 15*, 285.

Tew, J., Ramon, S., Slade, M., Bird, V., Melton, J., & Le Boutillier, C. (2012). Social factors and recovery from mental health difficulties: A review of the evidence. *The British Journal of Social Work, 42*(3), 443–460.

Warner, R. (2010). Does the scientific evidence support the recovery model? *The Psychiatrist, 34*(1), 3–5.

Zalsman, G., Hawton, K., Wasserman, D., van Heeringen, K., Arensman, E., Sarchiapone, M., … Zohar, J. (2016). Suicide prevention strategies revisited: 10-year systematic review. *The Lancet Psychiatry, 3*(7), 646–659.

Chapter 4
Expanding the Options Through Nine Steps

Contents

Amber's Recovery Pathway

I had just delivered my speech on the results of our SC2.0 Demonstration Project. The Minister of Health had opened the event by describing the Province's recently adopted "Towards Recovery" mental health strategy. The CEO of the Mental Health Commission of Canada spoke prior to me, sharing comments about how the project fits within a pan-Canadian context. Amber was invited up right after me. I had never met Amber and had no idea what she was planning to say. It turns out that I couldn't have scripted a better testimonial to the value of our nine-step model of care. She began by saying that she was a 23-year-old recent graduate from Memorial University and that this was the first time she had ever talked publicly about her mental illness. Despite this, she showed no signs of anxiety and the audience was soon riveted by her story. Amber recalled having severe bouts of anxiety and panic symptoms since in kindergarten. Years later, with her mental health deteriorating, she frequently cried herself to sleep. During the day she masked her panic with lies. One time a teacher asked why she was so out of breath, "Oh, I just went for a run on my lunch break". Ashamed and embarrassed, she was afraid to tell anyone about her weakness. In grade 11, Amber called Canada's Kids Help Phone. This was her first contact with the mental health system. The staff at Kids Help Phone were supportive, "They gave me the courage to finally tell my parents", she said. Amber's parents helped her connect with their family physician. Amber remembers her physician as kind, gentle and reassuring: "Amber, we're going to get you some help. It

P. Cornish, *Stepped Care 2.0: A Paradigm Shift in Mental Health*,
https://doi.org/10.1007/978-3-030-48055-4_4

is really good that you decided to talk about this with me and your parents". Amber replied sharply, "I don't want any meds!" She wasn't sure why at the time, just knew that they were a no-go. Much later, after a lot of self-reflection and support from CHANNAL (a local community-based peer network), she understood that it had to do with her values and personality. "I guess I have always been a stubborn person. I wanted to tackle the problem myself. I didn't want to change who I am or see myself as someone with a mental illness. I wanted to fight the problem myself". But at the time, neither Amber nor her physician knew quite how to proceed. She was referred for counselling. Amber was reluctant and nervous, Amber fought through the anxiety and doubts. She went for the counselling appointment. She was asked questions about her symptoms, her experiences of panic and the frequent night-time crying. Then, somewhat stunned, she heard the counsellor say something that threw her off, "Amber, you are being a dramatic teenager and you will get over it".

Amber was crushed. She retreated, gave up on help-seeking. There were no other options for counselling in her small community. Depression took over. "Depression", she said, "it was sort of like having four or five of those blackout curtains wrapped tightly around my whole body. I couldn't see a thing. I couldn't move. What was happening? I would feel hot and clammy, followed by chills. I couldn't move. I was alone and trapped with my negative, despairing thoughts".

There wasn't a dry eye in the room at this point. I heard someone crying softly behind me. Amber's speech, I noticed turning my head to the left, was being recorded. The young woman holding up the smart phone just behind me had tears streaming down her face. Later while watching the recording, I could hear the suppressed sobs and a few sniffles from Amber's younger sister. At that moment in her speech, Amber acknowledged her sister and said if it wasn't for her, she may not be alive.

Both family and peer support were essential for Amber's recovery, "I was in my third year of university when I got placed at CNIB (Canadian Institute for the Blind) for my first work term. CNIB works out of the same building as CHANNAL (the province-wide peer support network), just upstairs. At this time in my life, I was not very open about my mental illness and was not yet diagnosed with depression—only an anxiety disorder. I had never heard of CHANNAL before and was curious. My coworkers at CNIB told me it was a mental health and addictions organization. Living with mental illness myself, I was intrigued. I decided to look up CHANNAL's Facebook page and do a little research. It sounded like an amazing place, but I was not in a healthy mindset to use their services - I still had a lot of shame. I kept tabs on their Facebook page".

Amber's mood worsened. Suicidal thoughts became more frequent and graphic. She imagined herself jumping off a familiar cliff at the top of Signal Hill. The urge became overwhelming when she and her boyfriend parked one day at the top of the hill. But, "It was the love I feel for my sister that stopped me from acting on the impulse to jump. It was the thought of my sister that led me to my Dad. Mom was away. I told Dad about my scare on Signal Hill, and then I went back to my Doctor". Again, with genuine compassion, her physician said, "Amber, we're going to get you help" and once more she gently, yet firmly, recommended counselling and medication. Amber was ready now to consider a variety of options including counselling and medication. Her physician had recently learned about some new resources that had been implemented through our project and suggested that Amber check out the Bridge the gApp online mental health services directory/portal.

Amber valued autonomy. She speculated that, "It was probably my shyness, my shame and stubbornness, along with my do-it myself attitude, that attracted me first to the online tools on the website. I tried the mindfulness app, but I couldn't concentrate at the time. I found the "Art Room" where other kids had posted photos of drawings. There were so many other young people posting anonymously about their own feelings of panic and despair. I was shocked. I guess I'm not really alone. My confidence boosted, I explored some of the other tools. Breathing Room inspired me, building my confidence further. I tried some online therapy modules and eventually returned to the mindfulness app. With some of these skills and growing confidence, I reached out to CHANNAL. I had started opening up more about my mental illness and was ready to get the help I needed and to let go of the shame I was holding".

Recovery and resilience depend on the availability of timely opportunities, "CHANNAL had posted a job. I couldn't believe the timing; it was almost like fate. I decided to apply and just give it my best shot. If I didn't get the job, at least I took a step forward in my recovery and a step towards CHANNAL. Fortunately, I got the job along with six other amazing people. I became part of a family with the 12-plus people that were already working there. The support and respect were incredible, and I knew I had found the job that was for me. I have been there for almost a year now and am so thankful for CHANNAL and its role in my recovery". Amber paused and said with a wry smile, "You know at CHANNAL they try to break you!" A few knowing chuckles across the room. "The peer training is very intensive. They challenge you to do so much self-reflection".

At the news conference, Amber emerged as a valued spokesperson for the power of peer support. Her speech has since been adapted into a video explaining the importance of co-design, peer support and lived experience for our recovery-oriented SC2.0 Model.

4.1 Recovery Step by Step

In true recovery fashion, Amber entered the care system in her own way. I wonder what would have happened to her if the Province of Newfoundland and Labrador had not adopted *the Towards Recovery* strategy. The SC.0 model in Newfoundland and Labrador allowed Amber to access the help she was ready for, right at the time she sought help. Unfortunately, the model was not in place the first time she went looking and her condition had worsened. At the beginning, the anxiety she experienced had been unpleasant and restricted her social functioning. The only services available at that time were counselling and medication. Neither proved a good match for her. When the counselling backfired, there was no opportunity to fail forward. *Towards Recovery* had not been conceived. SC2.0 did not exist. Amber became severely depressed and suicidal. Luckily, according to Amber herself,

"Having a much wider selection of options available to me the second time I went to my doctor probably saved my life!" Amber's recovery could now proceed step by step.

4.2 How Many Steps Should There Be?

A review of published studies on stepped care reveals wide variability in the number of step categories. We were surprised to discover that the most common number of steps was only two. Our version, SC2.0 has the greatest number of steps. This is deliberate. We were interested in breaking care down into its most basic, elemental components. To our knowledge, the categories are exhausted at nine steps. Originally, we specified eight steps, but stakeholder input from one of our co-design implementation workshops led us to break psychoeducational and family/peer support into separate categories. Psychoeducation, we were told, could be delivered by either peers or professionals, or even both at the same time, in the form of workshops.

We believe that a high specificity of step levels maximizes the potential of stepped care. It encourages the discovery of ever more mental health resource options. With more options, comes greater potential for accommodating help seeker preference and maximizing treatment fit.

The most basic two-step model, formerly known as "shared care", has been around for decades. It typically involves transitioning back and forth between physician and psychiatric care. A more recent two-step model involves stepping between e-mental health and traditional face-to-face psychotherapy. Neither of these stepped care approaches would have worked for Amber. Face-to-face counselling, poorly timed for the state Amber was in at the time, was a setback for her. It was unhelpful and Amber lacked the confidence at the time to give this feedback to her physician. She dropped out of that treatment.

In the context of our SC2.0 model, Amber made use of five of the nine steps, only one of which existed several years ago. And while research suggests that individual psychotherapy and pharmacotherapy are highly effective for treating anxiety or depression (Cuijpers et al., 2013), it fails to account for barriers to access. Barriers to access for Amber included internalized stigma and lack of readiness to engage fully in the therapeutic process. Another barrier stemmed from the one-size-fits-all approach to psychotherapy referrals. The counsellor she had been referred to was not a good fit. There was no alignment or connection. Amber experienced the counsellor as dismissive. In a recovery-based SC2.0 context, Amber would have had more choice. She could have attended the same-day walk-in clinic. She would have known from the information in the waiting room, that choice was paramount. She would have known that if she didn't feel comfortable with her first experience, she could walk in another day and try someone else.

Amber's journey began with a Step-9 consultation. She reached out to Kids Help Phone; a crisis line staffed by professional counsellors. This worked for Amber because it removed an access barrier. It was easy for Amber to connect without anyone knowing. She made the call in the safety and privacy of her own bedroom. The help-line counsellor recommended a Step-3 resource—family support. She was nudged to open up to a loved one. Perhaps this worked because Amber made the call from a safe and relaxed place. She was ready to receive this recommendation. Family support was key to Amber's recovery. Her parents supported her to reach out to their family physician. This is a Step-7 resource—flexible individual professional support.

In Canada, physicians and psychiatrists are the only professionals that can bill directly the publicly funded Medicare system for counselling. This was the only accessible option known to Amber and her family at the time. The compassionate mental healthcare she received from her physician was critically important, but it was not enough. Amber needed more options. There were only two to choose from the first time—medication, or "talk therapy" with the one and only counsellor in her small community. There was no system aimed at empowering help-seekers. There was no encouragement to engage in trial and error among a variety of options. There was no buffet to sample from.

4.3 Step 1: Watchful Waiting; Informational Self-Directed

The second time she reached out, again through a Step-3 resource—family support, the mental health system in the Province had evolved. The Provincial *Towards Recovery* strategy had being launched (Government of Newfoundland and Labrador, 2017). There was a new mind-set among providers. Help-seeker preference was now emphasized and many more options were available. Amber's physician told her about the new and powerful Step-1 resource, Bridge the gApp. Step 1 focuses on information. It is aimed at supporting mental health literacy. Mental health literacy includes knowing the difference between distress and mental illness. Bridge the gApp is a mental health literacy site designed to educate. In order to be effective, the information at Step 1 must be evidence-informed and practical. It must include up-to-date resources, including a directory of programs available locally. It also should include details on how to access evidence-informed online resources. Bridge the gApp is such a resource. It is managed by mental health professionals and meets the highest privacy standards. It includes a directory of services organized by region. The directory includes both (1) formal, professionally and peer-led, publicly funded programs and (2) informal programs available in the community. Formal programs include counselling, psychological and psychiatric services as well as programming offered by paid, trained peer support workers. Formal programming also includes online tools funded by the government and available to all citizens free of charge. Informal programs include community-based programs and support groups such as AA, NA, Big Sisters and Brothers and Survivors of Suicide.

Step 1 also includes the notion of "watchful waiting". Amber's physician referred her to *Bridge the gApp* after learning of Amber's bad experience with counselling and she already knew that Amber did not want medication. She wasn't sure if Amber was ready to try the new walk-in, single-session counselling program called "Doorways". Amber's preference and/or readiness for engaging in intensive programming was unclear. As such, her physician simply prescribed Step 1: Self-directed informational resources and watchful waiting. Step 1 can be a good option when readiness is low or preferences hard to determine. Watchful waiting in the context of SC2.0 involves no specific recommendation, but instead an agreement to keep an eye on things through continued wellness monitoring. Research suggests this, alone, can be an effective intervention with at least 20% of help-seekers recovering after making an initial contact and receiving no specific treatment (Whiteford et al., 2012). When watchful waiting is prescribed along with access to solid, accessible mental health literacy tools, this percentage may well increase.

Amber spent a lot of time at Step 1. She discovered and experimented with a variety of resources available through the *Bridge the gApp* portal. From that vantage point, she moved up and down from Step 2 (interactional self-directed resources) and Step 3 (peer support). Step 1 proved to be a safe harbour for Amber. It laid the foundation for her to experiment with options, to sample the buffet, to risk trial and error. Her first attempt at the Step-2 *MindWell* app was a failure. It required too much concentration. She was too easily distracted at that time. No matter; the *Art Wall* was there. Colouring calmed her. Reading what peers posted helped her to fight internal stigma. She felt less alone with her symptoms. She kept exploring and trying out the various Step-1 options and, as her mental health literacy grew, she made progress with recovery.

4.4 Step 2: Interactive Self-Directed

Step 2 requires a little more commitment and energy than Step 1. The assumption at this step is that a help-seeker will become a more active and committed learner. Programming at Step 2 moves beyond mental health literacy. It calls for sustained participation. The participation at Step 2 is private. It typically involves completing workbooks or worksheets. These can be paper-based or online. Prior to the internet, this was referred to as bibliotherapy—self-help treatment with a book or workbook. One popular example of bibliotherapy is David Burn's book, *Feeling Good: The New Mood Therapy* (Burns, 1981). This is a cognitive behavioural therapy self-help manual. Ironically, this was the text we had proposed to use in our failed self-help study described in the preface to this book. We estimated that the book had been written at a grade six reading level, but we underestimated the extent to which reading *books* had become unpopular. In hindsight, I wonder if the study may have succeeded were *Bridge the gApp* and some online Step-2 programs had been available? After all, *online* reading is now the preferred medium.

Amber accessed several Step-2 resources. The first one she tried was *MindWell U*. This is a 30-day mindfulness course. It requires a minimum of 3–5 min of work per day. Each day, participants receive an email from *MindWell* with a link to the day's unique content, along reminders and tips on how to practice the *Take-5* meditation (see Fig. 4.1 for description of the Take-5 exercise). The programming is dynamic and has a well-designed user-interface. In other words, it is attractive, enticing and easy to use. To encourage commitment, users can select a "buddy"—a friend or family member—who they can invite to register for the program. Users are encouraged to connect with their buddies to share experiences, encourage each other or engage in some friendly competition around participation goals. With this buddy feature, *MindWell* has an element of a Step-3 program (peer support).

Although intrigued by the program—she had set herself a goal of becoming more relaxed through mindfulness meditation—Amber decided the program was not right for her at the time. She couldn't concentrate enough to follow the Take-5 meditation exercise, which was central to the program. Instead, she found the *TAO* program, with its more basic relaxation tools, a better fit with her capacities. Whereas, *MindWell* prescribed scheduled fixed content for each of the 30 days of the program, the *TAO* self-managed program allowed more flexibility. Amber was able to browse the modules, picking and choosing programming corresponding with her readiness. She found that the simple relaxation training exercises in *TAO* required less concentration than the Take-5 mindfulness protocol. A screenshot for one of the TAO modules on relaxation is illustrated in Fig. 4.2.

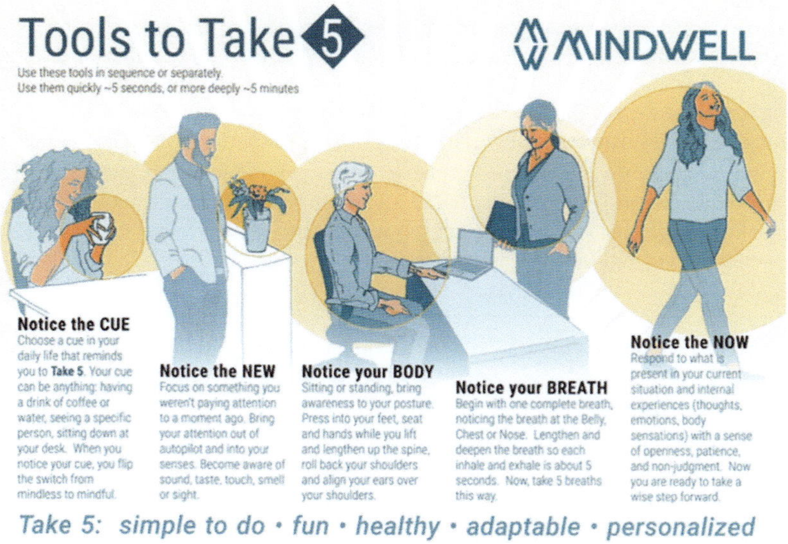

Fig. 4.1 Mindwell U's Take-5 mediation exercise (Mindwell, 2020)

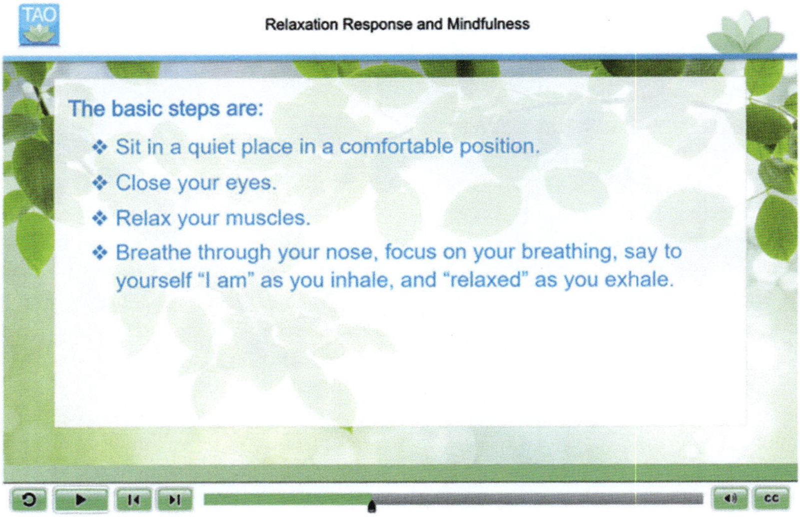

Fig. 4.2 TAO Connect's mindfulness module screenshot

4.5 Step 3: Family and Peer Support

When Amber contacted *Kids Help Phone* line (Step 9), the crisis counsellor listened to her concerns and encouraged her to reach out to her parents for support. This was a good example of an effective *stepping down* intervention. The help-line counsellor sensed Amber was not ready or unable to access professional care but had a good relationship with her parents. Reaching out to her parents was a simple, elegant option. She was ready and willing to do this. Family support was the home base for Amber's attempts to access formal professional care. Without Step 3, Amber would not have accessed the range of resources she needed.

While not understood as such, Amber already had engaged in Step-3 support. Specifically, her connection with her younger sister and her parents are examples of *informal*, unpaid community-based peer support. *Formal* peer support, in contrast, is typically paid work which requires standardized training, supervision and certification. The type of informal family and peer support offered through organizations like AA is voluntary and includes little or no training or oversight. Both are valuable. Amber said that she probably would not be alive if it wasn't for her love for her younger sister.

After her failed attempt with professional counselling and her successful work with self-managed e-mental health tools (at Steps 1 and 2), Amber discovered the formal peer support network, CHANNAL. Amber certainly valued her autonomy and the informal supports extended by her family. It is perhaps no surprise then that formal peer support was a logical step up when she became ready. She needed more than informal support but found professional care (talk therapy and medication) too intense initially, the dosage of care was too high. Formal peer support was skill-based (the peers who supported her had received certified paraprofessional training). It also included access to a community of peers, as well as a welcoming physical space (like a clubhouse). This formal peer support enabled stable connection that was also empowering. Amber initially felt uncomfortable being in the passive position of simply *receiving* treatment. She saw herself as strong, a fighter and someone who finds meaning and purpose through giving to others. Amber probably does not realize how much she has already given to others. By sharing her story publicly, in front of television cameras, the Minister of Health and other local and national dignitaries, Amber has proven the untapped power and potential for peer support to empower people while also reforming our mental health system.

4.6 Step 4: Workshops

Step 4 is the first point on the care continuum where professionals may enter the picture. Unlike group counselling or therapy, the focus in Step-4 workshops is mainly educational; it does not typically involve disclosure or much interaction among attendees. The format is akin to a class or presentation. While there are some similarities to Step 1, insofar as the aim is increasing mental health literacy, the commitment and energy required by both attendees and presenters are typically greater. For an attendee, there is a social commitment to stay for at least an entire session. It involves some public exposure. Others will know of the attendee's interest, thereby compromising privacy. However, unlike group therapy, participants will not learn much more than that. There is little chance of sensitive information being revealed. This can make it feel safe.

In a few of the communities where we implemented SC2.0, workshops were the most popular option. For example, on the Burin Peninsula, a region experiencing a rash of suicides a few years ago, workshops on mood and anxiety fill to capacity. This may be a logical extension of the successful community lobbying efforts that fast-tracked the Provincial *Towards Recovery* rollout (Government of Newfoundland and Labrador, 2017). Community members had already discovered power in numbers. They had achieved much through town hall meetings following the suicides. That attending workshops together might continue to foster mental health was a no-brainer; they already knew the healing power of community.

4.7 Step 5: Guided Self-Help

Guided self-help is a little like the so-called "flipped classroom". A flipped classroom is a post-secondary course modality that blends human contact with web-based content. High-quality content is procured and offered asynchronously through web-based video and interactive programming. Presentations by some of the world's most gifted educators can be recorded and accessed online anytime by students. Typically, weekly interaction with a tutor or instructor is scheduled. This face-to-face, classroom-based, interaction focuses on problem-solving, answering questions and motivating task completion. While flipped classrooms have demonstrated proof of concept (i.e. learning does occur), widespread implementation has not happened (O'Flaherty & Phillips, 2015). They account for a very small percentage of post-secondary curriculum delivery (McPherson & Bacow, 2015).

With Step-5 mental healthcare, the guided sessions can be in person, online or in group format. The focus may include technology troubleshooting, motivational interviewing to maximize module engagement, or addressing gaps arising from other mental health needs. Guided self-help has demonstrated very impressive results through clinical trials—almost always matching the outcomes achieved by traditional face-to-face 50-min weekly psychotherapy sessions but using far less professional time and expense (Andersson et al., 2014). However, much like flipped classrooms, guided self-help just hasn't caught on. In both cases, practitioners are unmotivated, or perhaps not well enough prepared, to adopt the new practice. Very little training is available to supply educators or therapists with knowledge or skills for successfully implementing web-based learning.

Rather than waiting for practitioners to adapt their practices to include technology, some clinic decision-makers are contracting out the work. A growing number of online psychotherapy platform developers have begun recruiting their own clinicians. Only those with interest in e-therapy work and grounding in recovery principles are considered for the positions. They are expected to specialize in this modality. Although there are no clear signs yet, this could mark the beginning of disruption in the mental health field akin to Uber's influence on the Taxi industry. Will therapists and their professions adapt or might they fall prey to some more massive, as yet unforeseen e-mental health disruption?

Currently, there are two types of vendors operating in the expert-assisted e-mental health space. Therapy-Assisted Online (known as TAO-Connect) was one of the first commercially available platforms. It is a social enterprise aimed at having a significant positive impact on campus mental health. Priced aggressively, it is easily absorbed through the limited budgets of college and university counselling centres. TAO provides the platform, a video conferencing function, a wide variety of transdiagnostic modules, and practice-based therapeutic measurement tools. TAO does not provide any labour. Clinics use their own professional staff. As such, counselling centres must somehow prepare and convince existing staff to adapt practices. This is proving to be very challenging. Few psychotherapists have shown interest. As such, companies like TAO Connect are adapting their business models by reaching outside clinic settings where there are more willing coaching partners. The shift means moving away from expert clinician guidance to peer or paraprofessional coaching. On campuses, residence leaders, athletics staff and judicial affairs officers have started to take this on. Some are prescribing the programming regularly now to the students they serve.

Mind Beacon is a Canadian startup that *is* succeeding with the expert-assisted e-mental health model. They recruit and train both psychologists and wellness advisors to support customers using their CBT platform which is designed to treat both anxiety and depression. While easier to implement because the therapists are supplied by the vendor, the program is expensive. Therapists are hired and trained specifically to support clients using the platform. This model addresses the key obstacle to implementing therapist-assisted e-mental health: professional change management. However, therapist involvement is not the only challenge. Purchasers of the solution still need to establish referral pathways and market the innovation to clients. While clinician training would not be required, stakeholder buy-in is needed to facilitate appropriate referrals and stepping decisions. Unfortunately, even with a strong evidence base supporting both guided (Andersson, Cuijpers, Riper, & Heidman, 2014) and self-guided (Karyotaki et al., 2017) e-mental health programming, providers remain largely unconvinced. That is, many believe few clients would either choose or benefit from anything other than face-to-face traditional 50-min weekly psychotherapy. However, since the onset of COVID-19 early in 2020, interest in these programs has increased. The pandemic is accelerating the shift to digital mental health.

A carefully designed change management program is needed to ensure Step-5 success. Training might include increasing provider technical proficiency, developing a coaching mind-set, and encouraging treatment adherence. Some clinics have succeeded by seconding early adopters to specialized implementation roles. With release from regular duties, they are able to focus energy on championing the program and mentoring colleagues. Some of these innovators found success in delivering the e-mental health client coaching component through a group counselling format. This has worked especially well in settings that routinely deploy two facilitators to lead groups. Such cases afford an opportunity for mentoring less enthusiastic colleagues. This apprenticeship approach could be a vehicle for gently nudging buy-in from therapists otherwise reluctant to offer guided e-mental health programming on their own.

4.8 Step 6: Intensive Group Programming

Group psychotherapy is a powerful and effective treatment modality; however, group has long played second fiddle to individual psychotherapy. Many mental health professionals see individual face-to-face psychotherapy as the gold standard treatment. Anything else short changes help-seekers. Like guided e-mental health programming, group psychotherapy is proven effective but underutilized. There are several explanations for this tendency to undervalue group psychotherapy. One is that therapists themselves say they would not opt for group therapy given a choice. Perhaps, this is because it is a high dosage treatment largely due to the social exposure element. Opening up to peers and being challenged by both peers and therapists in a closed environment is not for the faint of heart. From a client perspective, group therapy might better be thought of as a higher intensity treatment than individual therapy. Currently, we situate group therapy at Step 6 just below individual therapy because from a funding perspective group requires less investment. Perhaps the order of the steps should be reversed for client-facing depictions of the model. Understandably, help-seekers may feel some trepidation when offered group psychotherapy. Consider a person struggling with social anxiety. Theoretically, we might argue group therapy is the treatment of choice. The group setting affords a safe place to fully experience, understand and develop skills for coping with anxiety. But client readiness and preference almost always trump theory. As such, it may not be the best place to start treatment.

The underutilization of group psychotherapy is also related to inadequate training. Typically, training in group therapy is limited by a relatively thin curriculum and sparse practicum site opportunities. Under such conditions, we cannot expect to develop a critical mass of confident group therapists needed to raise the profile, legitimacy and availability of this powerful modality.

Nevertheless, SC2.0 training and implementation help motivated providers to develop a variety of alternatives to the Step-7 gold standard. An incremental approach to group program development, in the context of this larger transformation process, holds promise. Without a lot of previous experience or training in group work, it is fair to assume inexperienced practitioners would not begin by facilitating open-ended process groups. Nor would they cut their teeth working with populations likely to challenge authority. Starting with highly structured groups makes a lot more sense. The structure allows leaders to maintain control. This is important for building confidence. Lecture and workshop psycho-educational formats, like those outlined above at Step 4, are the most structured types of groups. Just as Amber needed to begin with low-intensity programming, therapists might need to begin with Step-4 practices before attempting the more intensive Step-6 work. At Step 4, communication is unidirectional, thereby precluding any need to manage interactions. In contrast, group psychotherapy at Step 6 is by nature more unpredictable. Group psychotherapy participants are often expected to display their maladaptive interpersonal patterns in vivo. Not a good experience for neophyte therapists. Quite often the most valuable learning for clients comes from working through authority issues by challenging the leadership. Few therapists are ready for this straight out of the gate. Some may never choose it.

For agencies and clinics that have decided to adopt SC2.0, not all steps are populated at once. Implementing a group therapy program in the context of SC2.0 is best done incrementally. If group work has not been a key part of the treatment continuum at a clinic, it would make sense to begin with structured educational approaches focusing on mental health literacy in Step 4. Perhaps the next step in implementation would be to move to semi-structured psychotherapy groups. These groups have well-developed curricula and are more akin to teaching a class. There is some interaction but the interaction is limited to the parameters of pre-set exercises. While there may be some open-ended disclosure and unstructured interactions, these are usually restricted by returning to the pre-set agenda of the sessions.

I suggest that the most highly structured therapy groups be classified as Step-4 interventions, whereas semi-structured psychotherapy groups are best categorized as either Step-6 or Step-8 interventions, depending on the client population. Groups specifically targeting clients with highly sensitive and interpersonally volatile presentations should be considered Step-8 specialist level interventions. A basic Yalom-style interpersonal process psychotherapy group is highly unstructured and as such it fits the category of intensive group work. This is by design. The lack of structure creates space, a social microcosm, whereby clients' maladaptive patterns can play out safely within the context of skilled group leadership. And depending on the volatility of the clients attending, this could be classified as either Step 6 or 8. In an outpatient clinic context, a Yalom-style group would be considered a Step 6 level intervention. Trauma groups or DBT groups in residential or inpatient settings would be classified as Step 8. Readiness for exposure and being challenged are key factors when considering referrals to groups at Steps 6 and 8.

Developing group programming can be frustrating. Groups require considerable upfront planning and some risk that this time will not pay off. Why put all the work into planning when participant recruitment is so challenging? Many practitioners report attempts at planning groups only to discover few people accept referrals. Scheduling is naturally more complicated by the fact that, even if willing and eligible clients were to be identified, it is likely that a time would not be found to accommodate all. Even if these challenges are met, repeated reluctance expressed by clients can be enough to discourage all attempts. This is understandable, particularly if groups offered never fill or have to be cancelled due to low numbers. Some providers, those with high caseloads or increasing demand, may persevere. Growing frustration may lead them to a hard sell approach, "I won't see you unless you go to group first". I do not expect much success with this approach unless the programming is well-matched to client readiness. Offering choices might help especially if a series of groups, with varying levels of structure or exposure intensity, are available.

Some theorists have emphasized the importance of group therapy preparation sessions or workshops. There is evidence that this increases attendance and outcomes (Piper & Perrault, 2015). There is certainly room in SC2.0 to offer group preparation at a lower level within the continuum of care. After all, readiness is a core variable in stepping decisions. If a clinic setting has a long wait time for individual therapy, clients may be open to attending a workshop entitled "Everything you would like to know about group therapy". Some may be enticed by this one-time information session and enrol in group therapy. Others might decide to wait. In both cases, offering the choice is empowering.

While readiness is a key factor in SC2.0, the goal of preparing people for higher level programming conflicts with a key principle of our model. Instead of moving people to a level that practitioners would like to practice, the goal in SC2.0 is to move the treatment to where the person is ready without any assumption that more is needed. Of course, a help-seeker may wish to strive for more and this is fine. But it is more empowering and less burdensome on the care system to leave the question of "Is this enough or should there be more" up to the help-seeker.

4.9 Step 7: Flexible Intensive Individual Programming

Step 7 is undoubtedly where most work currently happens in mental healthcare. While the demand can be reduced with the implementation of SC2.0, social workers, psychologists, counsellors, physicians, nurses and psychiatrists will continue to deliver some form of talk therapy on a routine basis. Often the style, complexity, duration and interval of treatment are different depending on the provider or discipline. This is a good thing, as one size does not fit all. Client preference and choice are core principles of SC2.0. However, there is considerable debate among providers and uncertainty among help-seekers about what to expect from whom.

In SC2.0, informed consent is especially important. This is partly because the model and approaches are new. It is also because having clear expectations improves outcomes. Equally important to informed consent is role clarity. This includes the expectations and roles of both client and provider, but increasingly in our more collaborative care networks, we need to do more to develop interprofessional role clarity. What should a nurse do in the SC2.0 system? What about the family physician, a psychiatrist or a psychologist? While we have not yet worked this out, the model does provide a kind of scaffolding for exploring and testing out role differentiation. This is detailed more in Chap. 6.

Have you ever wondered why psychotherapists typically work in the context of the 50-min hour? This has been the case for more than a century. An hour is a useful period of time for costing. An hourly rate is easily understood and remains the most common unit for pricing all wages in our economy. The extra 10 min afforded by the 50-min hour, of course, ensures that time spent with record keeping and other administrative tasks are factored into the pricing. But what does science say about this? Is this unit of time any better than others for improving mental health? And then, what about weekly intervals, why do we practice psychotherapy at one-week intervals? Is there evidence to support this? Is the weekly 50-min session in the best interest of help-seekers or is it really for providers? Of course, we do need a system that is sustainable. The needs of providers are important, but they should not preclude innovation.

Very little research has addressed these questions. That in itself is interesting. Why hasn't this been studied more? The research that has been conducted suggests that there is nothing particularly beneficial or important about intervals and session duration (Erickson, Lambert, & Eggett, 2015; Turner, Valtierra, Talken, Miller, & DeAnda, 1996). While it is true that much more study is warranted before drawing firm conclusions, proponents of SC2.0 encourage more experimentation in general and this also applies to the use of time. In the context of continuous therapeutic measurement, client preference and a trial and error philosophy, therapists operating at Step 7 can become much more creative with time. Sometimes we ask our clients at the beginning of Step-7 sessions, "What would you prefer today, a targeted brief 15-min skill-building session or a longer meeting to explore and dig deeper? Do you want to get something done today or delve into understanding the complexity of your life?"

With a client who is exhausted due to lack of sleep, or one with low energy levels associated with depression, maybe a briefer session is in order. With what little energy there is, a shorter, more focused session could be more productive. For someone who finds the sessions highly anxiety provoking, a small dosage might be more tolerable. My colleagues who work with indigenous peoples sometimes suggest a day-long session on the land makes far more sense than seven or eight 50-min meetings.

My life partner, Karen, is an experienced psychologist who owns and operates a small private practice. She is known in the community for her experience in treating complex cases, including clients with Borderline Personality Disorder, Bipolar Disorder and Complex PTSD. She sees her clients more regularly and for longer periods than I do. As I was finishing writing this book, we were beginning preparations for an international move. This meant that Karen was considering how to terminate treatment with her clients. She received an email request for therapy from a person with a long and complex history of mental illness. She was working on a response and asked me for advice on what to say in the email. I asked what her concern was. She replied, "I am not sure how I should indicate that I will only be practicing here for the next six months". I asked her why she thought that was necessary. She answered, "Well, if I don't tell the client then she won't be able to make an informed choice about whether to see me for such a short time". I said, "But if you do tell her in advance, aren't you subtly implying that six months might not be enough for her? How does that instill hope?"

Some colleagues, including my partner Karen, say to me, "Surely there is value in a course of 10–20 (or more) 50-min sessions for those people with complex needs, such as complex PTSD". I agree that this might be helpful but suggest it need not be the default. Why not be more flexible? Why not ask the help-seeker? "But", say may colleagues, "It can take a long time for someone who has been abused for years to build up trust in a therapist. Having briefer and fewer sessions would further delay this process". This may be true for some, but then I question aren't there many ways to build trust? Colleagues sometimes counter with, "You can't rush the development of the therapeutic bond. This happens very slowly". While there is a large and robust body of research underscoring the value of the therapeutic alliance in driving mental health outcomes, the alliance does not necessitate a deep and lasting bond. Our goal is not to replicate friendship. Such an effort would be considered unethical for a variety of reasons—creation of dependency, profiting through the dependency, doing more harm than good. Instead the alliance is about alignment. Alignment can happen within a matter of seconds. A gifted health practitioner does this frequently. Think of a talented and beloved rural family physician. With kind eyes and a warm, gentle smile, such a physician aligns swiftly and smoothly with patients. I call this "flash empathy". Unfortunately, we have not given enough attention to teaching alignment. Without adequate training, we are left waiting patiently with our clients for it to develop slowly and naturally over the course of many sessions.

With SC2.0, we do not dawdle when it comes to connecting. Professional development on forming rapid connection is a must. The model requires swift alignment with a therapeutic success in every encounter. With SC2.0, we remind ourselves of the fact that an initial encounter is likely to be the one and only. Even if a course of sessions is contracted at Step 7, we work hard to align anew each time, just in case it may be the last.

I now practice most of my psychotherapy one-session-at-a-time. I have many clients, most of whom I see infrequently. While not nearly the same number, this is akin to a typical family physician who has a large roster of patients, most of whom do not need medical attention. Some clients I see only once or twice. I believe they get what they came for. Because I have shared with them principles of the SC2.0 model, including start-strong/start-simple, trial and error, fail forward and come back if/when needed, clients begin feeling empowered and reassured that care is there when they need it. This produces rapid alignment. Sometimes I say, "I will work really hard today to make sure that you walk away feeling like this was helpful, that we did something useful and that something has already been achieved. But if, tomorrow, you think we might have missed something or got it wrong today, I really would like you to come back". This does two things related to alignment. The fact that I promise to work really hard to make sure that something therapeutic happens right away instils hope, optimism and faith in me as a dedicated helper. Secondly, a help-seeker does not feel pressured to get everything right, to solve all their problems right now, because they know they can come back. I often invite clients to think of visiting me in the same way they visit their family physician. Come when you need to. I will be available. Because my dominant form of practice is therapy one-at-a-time, I can usually accommodate requests for sessions within a week or two. Sometimes, when there is energy and substantial momentum, we may commit to a run of weekly sessions. Regardless of the pace or frequency, we review progress using therapeutic measurement at every session to guide treatment planning. If the data indicate deterioration or flattening of progress, we might decide together to experiment with adjusting the modality, frequency or duration of contacts.

Sometimes with people whom I have followed for longer than average, I make use of the traditional assessment, diagnostic and therapeutic techniques I was trained in. But I do this only when we are both feeling puzzled or stuck. The results can be spectacular and the outcome rewarding for both me and the client. In other cases, we discover through the use of therapeutic measurement and the successful reapplication of solution-focused interviewing, that a return (or stepping down) to periodic, one-at-a-time sessions is preferred. In a case where outcomes are flat or deteriorating, we will re-examine the treatment plan and consider the many other options available along the SC2.0 continuum. Some clients do initially experience stepping down as a threat to the connection we have established. If so, I liken it to a family physician's responsibility to find allied care options, to refer to specialists, to recommend strategies for lifestyle changes. In other words, I remind clients that I am still available to them, but I will not see myself as the only healer. I can be your touchpoint, your mental health go-to-consultant in the way that a family physician considers their clinic as the patients' medical home. In similar fashion, at Step 7, in SC2.0, the provider takes on the role of mental health treatment coordinator, or their mental healthcare treatment home.

4.10 Step 8: Chronic Care and Specialist Consultation

Consultation is an area for growth within the context of SC2.0. There is a need for our most highly trained, expensive mental health practitioners to work to their full scope of practice. While there are decades of research supporting the efficacy of talk psychotherapy, there is very little evidence indicating that level of training, discipline or years of practice reliably influence outcomes (Boswell, Castonguay, & Wasserman, 2010; Stein & Lambert, 1995). In other words, a social worker with a year of post-graduate training is typically about as effective as a psychologist or psychiatrist with 6 years of post-graduate training. There is a perception that professions with more years of training provide better psychotherapy. This has led funders (insurance companies and government funded Medicare plans) to authorize payments to providers that are the most expensive and potentially no more effective. Secondly, it allows specialists to do basic psychotherapy work that less costly providers could do. Not only is this inefficient, but it also means that specialists are not working to full scope. Both psychiatrists and psychologists working to full scope would prioritize more consultation and assessment for complex cases by either treating the complex cases themselves or advising generalist practitioners on treatment plans.

If mental health specialists were working to full scope, their practices would have greater resemblance to those of medical specialists such as urologists, oncologists and internists. For these specialty groups, the ongoing "contract" is with the general practitioner who receives their reports. The patient is only a client to the specialist for the one episode of care. The primary care physician is the specialist's true client. Unlike other medical specialists, mental health specialists (including psychiatrists and psychologists) often carry cases for long periods of time without discharging back to their medical home—the primary care physician. Without evidence suggesting that long-term care by mental health specialists is any better than support by lower intensity providers, this type of expensive practice is both inefficient and unethical.

Some of my psychiatrist and psychologist colleagues are reluctant to move completely into consultation roles. This is understandable. They were trained to work long-term directly with help-seekers and to value the development of a therapeutic bond. Part of what makes the work rewarding is the maintenance of these bonds over time and the fact that work with patients tends to become easier as they become known to providers. Both the patients and the providers become more relaxed through familiarity. My colleagues argue that burnout could increase if they only worked with the most complex cases or lost opportunities to form more comfortable alliances with patients. This is possible, but only if other rewards are not in place. I can think of two possible incentives. First a consulting role should be valued more, and payments should be higher. Secondly, practices should be set up so that the relationships formed are with the other professionals benefitting from their consultation.

One simple way to cultivate these relationships is through the development of integrated wellness hubs. These hubs could exist in both primary and tertiary care settings. Currently, specialists are not usually aligned with either primary or tertiary care settings. Most often, specialists work in private practice or acute care settings. Neither of these settings allow for specialists to maximize the impact of their consultation expertise. While specialist work may be essential for treatment of complex disorders, private practice care tends to prolong care longer than is necessary. The impact of specialist care in acute care settings is limited by the restricted healing capacity of patients that are in hospital mainly to be stabilized. Complex treatments that have the potential to impact recovery do not usually begin until after stabilization.

4.11 Step 9: Acute Care, Systems Navigation, Case Management and Advocacy

In the context of SC2.0, treatment at Step 9 expands to include more meaningful partnerships with both formal and informal community-based organizations. This is needed to improve care transitions, ensure follow-up by the right provider, and reduce frustrations and inefficiencies associated with the emergency department revolving door syndrome. Many people in crisis attend emergency departments when in high distress because there are no other real or perceived options. As a result, those in high distress who are not acutely ill (i.e. do not require psychiatric stabilization) are either not admitted or are discharged quickly. This is reasonable, given that the purpose of acute care is to save lives and stabilize. It is not aimed at recovery work or complex treatment.

With the development of lower step programming, including open access modalities on first contact, inappropriate mental health presentations at the emergency department can be reduced substantially. When peer support programming is available for people in distress (but not suicidal), emergency visits are also decreased. In Newfoundland and Labrador, CHANNAL operates clubhouse drop-in centres in various locations across the province. They also staff a peer-supported "Warmline". In contrast to crisis help lines, the Warmline offers supportive, active listening to people who are not in crisis. It is staffed by persons with lived experience of mental illness who have received intensive, certified peer-support training. Included in the Warmline brief assessment protocol is a question asked at the end of the phone call, "If this service were not available, what would you have done today?" In many cases callers indicate that they would have visited the emergency department.

Trained peer support workers are increasingly valued on hospital wards for their discharge planning and facilitation work. Not only is this work being done in psychiatric wards, but increasingly people with lived experience are facilitating social and mental health adjustment for patients discharged from oncology and cardiology words. They are also helping with adjustment in chronic disease management, facilitating early discharge without risking rebound admissions attributed to inadequate community supports.

Case management teams are becoming more common at various levels throughout the care continuum. Nurses or social workers are typically tasked with managing or coordinating the teamwork. These teams often include community stakeholders and trained peer supporters. Coordinators offer supervision and advice to team members. The coordinators likewise develop community-wide networks with counterparts operating at various levels of care. For example, almost every post-secondary institution now has a case management team. The case managers may operate within wellness clinics or independently. Team members include heads of counselling, the health clinic, accessibility services, campus police, residence life, the international students' office and academic advising. The coordinator's job is twofold: (1) to support team members in making appropriate care referrals and (2) in cases where referrals are not needed, to advise on how to maintain informal community support. For example, an accessibility advisor may get direction at a team meeting on coaching a student's supervisor in active listening techniques for moments when their student is in distress.

Case managers function as both system navigators and healthy community development advisors. This dual role has the potential to reduce or reverse the hot-potato referral tendency that has arisen within the context of the risk paradigm dominating both our care and judicial processes.

Within acute care settings, case managers coordinate care transitions required upon discharge. In the context of SC2.0 hospital-based case managers form partnerships with community-based case managers and care navigators. For example, in the City of Halifax in Nova Scotia, case managers in hospital settings have formed an alliance with the city's ten post-secondary institutions through a program called "Stay Connected". They rotate regular meeting locations across institutions so that case managers become familiar with the types of care offered along the stepped care continuum at the various sites. This has allowed them to develop efficient referral pathways and maintain coordinated care without duplication and while minimizing loss of continuity in care.

SC2.0 can only work if all parties are familiar with the whole system of care. Given that the system is dynamic—always in a state of evolution or improvement—it is difficult to see the forest for the trees. System navigators and case managers attend to this dialectic. They have eyes on the moving parts, can help with treatment planning and life-transitions on the micro level, but are also crucial partners, at the macro level, in system design and adjustment. They focus in and out on parts and system. Increasingly, people with lived experience with mental illness participate in this design work under supervision of case managers. In some cases, client design teams dedicated to system adjustment are established. For example, at Memorial University in 2017 we launched our first client design team. As described in the story at the end of Chap. 5, our design team was comprised of students with either lived experience of mental illness or an interest in improving care at the University. The team was led by a graduate student in educational psychology who, in turn, was supervised by our case manager. They worked over the course of a year to research, report and recommend feasible improvements and adjustments to our stepped care model. They presented this to the wellness clinic operations manager at the end of the academic year. Almost all recommendations were implemented. This design work, involving people familiar with various levels of the care continuum and supervised by case managers who can see the forest for the trees, ensures that care coordination and innovation are one and the same. It also elevates the recovery principle of empowerment through all levels of SC2.0.

Knit and Talk

When we made our first SC2.0 training site visit to the small Newfoundland coastal community of Lewisporte, we invited the clinicians and mangers in attendance to populate the nine steps in our model with existing programs available in their region. Using a white board, we began by drawing the x- and y-axes to represent the two dimensions of the model: Stakeholder investment on the y-axis and program intensity/client autonomy on the x-axis. We then created boxes and labelled each along the diagonal. The task for the group exercise was to "populate the steps" above and below the boxes. By this we explained that programs existing within clinic settings should be arranged under the appropriate step boxes and resources existing external to the clinic (both formal and informal) should be listed above the boxes. Programs below the diagonal included "Doorways" walk-in appointments at Step 1, "choice appointments" at Step 7, TAO programming at Steps 2 (self-managed TAO) and 5 (therapist assisted). Formal programs external to the clinic included, Strongest Families anxiety treatment program at Step 5 (this is delivered through contracting out telephone counselling to therapists located in another province), the Warmline (at Step 3) operated by the Province's peer support network and the Crisis Text Line (Step 9) operated by a non-profit national peer support network based in Toronto. We asked if there were any informal community supports that could be included above the line. Without delay we heard three voices in unison: "Knit and Talk". This women's support group had existed in the community for more than 20 years. While none of the clinicians had first-hand experience with the group, the reputation was positive. We asked if it should be included on the white board as a possible referral destination. Without hesitation the clinicians agreed. I asked, "What about liability, what if something goes wrong at Knit and Talk and someone you refer has a negative experience?" One of the more eager participants replied, "We are so past that now, Peter. We are not so risk averse. Besides we empower our clients to take managed risks, to fail forward when necessary, and we monitor outcomes regularly to ensure care is adjusted when necessary".

References

Andersson, G., Cuijpers, P., Riper, H., & Heidman, E. (2014). Guided Internet-based vs. face-to-face cognitive behavior therapy for psychiatric and somatic disorders: A systematic review and meta-analysis. *World Psychiatry, 13*(3), 288–295.

Boswell, J. F., Castonguay, L. G., & Wasserman, R. H. (2010). Effects of psychotherapy training and intervention use on session outcome. *Journal of Consulting and Clinical Psychology, 78*(5), 717–723.

Burns, D. D. (1981). *Feeling good: The new mood therapy*. New York: Penguin Books.

Cuijpers, P., Sijbrandij, M., Koole, S. L., Andersson, G., Beekman, A. T., & Reynolds, C. F. (2013). The efficacy of psychotherapy and pharmacotherapy in treating depressive and anxiety disorders: A meta-analysis of direct comparisons. *World Psychiatry, 12*(2), 137–148.

Erickson, D. M., Lambert, M. J., & Eggett, D. L. (2015). The relationship between session frequency and psychotherapy outcome in a naturalistic setting. *Journal of Consulting and Clinical Psychology, 83*(6), 1097–1107.

Government of Newfoundland and Labrador. (2017). *Towards recovery: A vision for a renewed mental health and addictions system for Newfoundland and Labrador.* St. John's: Government of Newfoundland and Labrador. Retrieved December 10, 2019, from https://www.health.gov.nl.ca/health/all_party_committe_report.pdf

Karyotaki, E., Riper, H., Twisk, J., Hoogendoorn, A., Kleiboer, A., Mira, A., ... Cuijpers, P. (2017). Efficacy of self-guided internet-based cognitive behavioral therapy in the treatment of depressive symptoms: A meta-analysis of individual participant data. *JAMA Psychiatry, 74*(4), 351–359.

McPherson, M. S., & Bacow, L. S. (2105). Online higher education: Beyond the hype cycle. *Journal of Economic Perspectives, 29*(4), 135–154.

Mindwell, U. (2020, January 4). *Take 5.* Retrieved from mindwellu.com: https://www.mindwellu.com/take-5

O'Flaherty, J. O., & Phillips, C. (2015). The use of flipped classrooms in higher education: A scoping review. *The Internet and Higher Education, 25*, 85–95.

Piper, W., & Perrault, E. L. (2015). Pretherapy preparation for group members. *International Journal of Group Psychotherapy, 39*(1), 17–34.

Stein, D. M., & Lambert, M. J. (1995). Graduate training in psychotherapy: Are therapy outcomes enhanced? *Journal of Consulting and Clinical Psychology, 63*(2), 182–196.

Turner, P. R., Valtierra, M., Talken, T. R., Miller, V. I., & DeAnda, J. R. (1996). Effect of session length on treatment outcome for college students in brief therapy. *Journal of Counseling Psychology, 43*(3), 228–232.

Whiteford, H. A., Harris, M. G., McKeon, G., Baxter, A., Pennell, C., Barendregt, J. J., & Wang, J. (2012). Estimating remission from untreated major depression: A systematic review and meta-analysis. *Psychological Medicine, 43*, 1569–1585.

Chapter 5
Navigating the System

Contents

Don't Step Me Down

"Don't give me any of that stepped care crap!" Lake had indeed read the consent form in the waiting room. The form described the stepped care model and what clients might expect. In the blank space for gender, Lake wrote "queer". I asked what pronouns Lake preferred and the response was "they/them". Lake explained that they had been highly suicidal and depressed throughout high school and the only thing that kept them alive was weekly 50-minute sessions with a therapist. "I don't want e-mental health apps and I don't want to go to a group". There was an edge to their voice, and I couldn't quite tell if it was anger, anxiety, or both. I thanked Lake for making this clear noting that client preference is really important to the kind of care we provide. "Tell me what was helpful about the work you did during high school," I asked. Lake replied, "Well, it kept me going. I was able to go to my classes, keep my parents off my back, and basically survive". "I'm glad to hear that", I said and asked, "What kinds of things did you and the therapist do during your sessions?" "I vented a lot. My therapist listened and supported me. I was able to get things off my chest and calm down. I don't think I would still be here if it wasn't for the therapy". Probing further, I said, "From the form you completed in the waiting room, I see that your symptoms of depression are still high and that you have thoughts of suicide a lot of the time". "Yes", Lake replied, "That's why I'm here". I asked Lake if they noticed any improvement in their mood or suicidal thoughts through the course of therapy. "Like I said, it kept me alive", Lakes patience was wearing thin. "And that is definitely a good thing. But, you know", I said, pausing for a moment, "I'm of two minds about this. I agree that staying alive is really important, but on the other hand, I'm wanting more for you than just surviving". Lake softened a little, looking puzzled. "What do you mean?" they asked. I

P. Cornish, *Stepped Care 2.0: A Paradigm Shift in Mental Health*,
https://doi.org/10.1007/978-3-030-48055-4_5

said, "When I work with clients, I do my best to go beyond managing symptoms. I work for growth, for wellness and I help clients to work hard for this too. Sometimes this doesn't happen right away, but I feel strongly that if I ask a person to come to weekly sessions, we are both going to do our best to make use of the time. My training goes beyond helping people to survive". Lake, frowning now, asked, "I'm not sure I understand. Not sure what that would look like to be working hard". I said, "We are doing it right now. I am challenging you to reach for wellness. You are puzzled, you are thinking hard, wondering what that would require from you". Lake responded, "I'm not sure I am comfortable with this. I work hard to keep alive. Isn't that enough?" "Well it could be enough. That's certainly an option. What I am saying is that if I were to work with you, that's what I expect. But we have other options if that doesn't feel right…" Lake interrupted, "I'm not doing anything online!" "No, while that is an option, there are many others", I said. "For example,we are a training site, and the graduate students working under our supervision are actually not allowed to challenge clients. Instead, their job is to listen and be supportive. I wonder if that is the kind of thing you are looking for?" Lake hesitated a moment and said, "As long as they won't send me to an app or a group". I said, "Not unless that is something to that would interest you".

5.1 Desire Pathways

SC2.0 is an open-access model with no pre-determined pathways. It is not a staging or pathways model. We do not purport to know in advance what pathways or levels of care would be appropriate for anyone. We also do not think a strict consultation process, whether through screening tools or formal assessments, is the best way to determine initial care approaches. To me, those would be like asking the architects to design the paths on a new campus, without consulting stakeholders. Instead, with SC2.0, we open up the field and point out the options and permit those who are interested to chart their course, seeking routes that make the most sense to them. Unlike other stepped care models, treatment need not be linear. There are many possible permutations and combinations of routes and reversals.

We always start with preference. Then, through some gentle probing, we get a sense of what intensity level can be tolerated. This leads to a reconsideration of preference. In other words, the preference is refined. How might this have looked for my daughter? We will never know because her preference was not assessed. As described in Chap. 2, my daughter had a negative experience with counselling. This happened twice. She went first to her university counselling centre and found the initial contact to be dominated by questions seemingly unrelated to her needs. She was offered an appointment 5 weeks later, but feeling discouraged by that initial disconnect, she declined. She assumed that paying out of pocket for a private practice session might ensure care more tailored to her needs with less waiting. Instead, she said the questions were the same. Neither counsellor ever asked what she wanted, or what she wanted to talk about. Instead, all questions were pre-determined.

My daughter admitted that she wasn't exactly sure what she needed. That is why she was seeking help. She did, however, know what her concerns were. Being asked 30 or 40 questions about things that were not a concern was frustrating. I agreed. I said, "It's like by turning over every stone, they will eventually discover some fascinating, deep dark mystery, and only then will you get help or relief". She said, "I knew what the problem was, I just wasn't sure about the solution".

I wonder how my daughter would have experienced SC2.0 programming. She is a freshly minted geologist with a passion for climate science. She, like many of her generation, was deeply distressed by the climate emergency facing our planet's inhabitants. She loves field work, the outdoors and does everything possible to avoid a desk.

With my amateur interest in architecture, I recently came across the concept of "desire pathways". These are pathways that evolve naturally without much forethought. Some urban planners have experimented on university campuses. No sidewalks or pathways are created when the campus first opens. Instead for a period of 6 months or so, designers observe where people naturally walk. They study the impressions left in the lawns or the gravel surrounding buildings. These are called desire pathways. If you leave space open for people to choose routes according to preference, what pathways would emerge? Once these become clear, contractors pave or otherwise reinforce the desired routes. Unfortunately, urban planners rarely consider this method.

I completed my predoctoral 12-month internship in psychology at a university in central Canada. I was struck upon my arrival by the lush, open green circular lawn in the middle of the campus. An interlocking brick path neatly marked the perimeter. Every 50 ft or so, a black wrought iron post topped with a gold letter sign warned pedestrians to "keep off the grass". The lawn was streaked with dusty, criss-crossing pathways allowing for expedient links among buildings.

Fall came quickly in this Northern city. Adding to this annual disappointment was the sudden appearance of a garishly bright orange snow fence—a temporary cross-hatched flimsy barrier, familiar to Northerners, designed to trap drifting snow. It was ugly, but at least only temporary. Winter in cities is often a dirty, messy affair. I was surprised to discover I was mistaken, when about a month later, construction began. The wrought-iron signs were replaced by a 4-ft-high iron fence. Forget desire pathways. There would be no pathways. Now everyone would be forced to follow the circuitous route year-round. What *was* the lush green lawn for anyway? What was the circle for?

I wonder if my daughter's experience of counselling was a little like that forced circuitous brick path. She had no choice but to follow someone else's ill-conceived path to get where they thought she should go. It was probably well-intentioned. Following protocols is meant to keep everyone safe. There will be no causalities or property damage. The lawn will remain pristine. It will control movement and prevent anyone from falling off the prescribed course.

But maybe she just needed to sit on the lawn for a while. After a while though, she would want to get going under her own steam. She thrives by finding her own path. Not only that, we need her and many others to chart new courses. The course prescribed by the last few generations now has the planet on suicide watch. Who are *we* to prescribe pathways? I think our expertise should pivot toward encouraging self-discovery and resilience, helping people find and stick to their preferred paths. They can always consult a chart or ask for help when lost. This is where our expertise with assessment can be recalibrated. Instead of a microscope or seismic drill designed to identify deep, dark structures below, our SC2.0 emphasis on therapeutic measurement is like a compass or a GPS device that can guide us to live productively on the Earth's surface where we do best.

I am a big believer in assessment. As a psychologist, I know that our tools for measuring, detecting and understanding complex pathology are powerful and can be very useful in formulating treatment plans. However, I think sometimes our approach to assessment is overpowered. Instead of a 200-horsepower turbo-charged engine, a bicycle or a pair of sturdy walking shoes might do. Maybe we could start with the shoes. A student like my daughter is moving under her own power. We start with trusting and believing that her description of the issue is correct until proven otherwise. We don't need to crush that self-propelled momentum that led to help-seeking with our turbo-charged psychometric tools. Instead, why not use our well-tested therapeutic measurement systems, our simple psychometric GPS, to see how well she creates her own paths. She could ask for help finding the path or she could consult a compass, map or GPS device. If progress is too slow, the wind too strong, we can assist and coach on solutions. We might even decide together that another route or mode of transport is needed. More sophisticated investigation, using more specialized diagnostic equipment might lead us to wonder if an e-bike kit would help or that public transit is the way to go. We might decide a full-sized vehicle, or one with a turbo-charged engine is needed after all for some travel. But going full-sized, without considering less energy-hungry options, is simply wasteful.

5.2 Open Navigation

If a patron samples a dish at a buffet that fails to meet expectations, they may return and try something else. Consumers decide themselves what they want with minimal direction. For a sit-down meal at an exclusive restaurant, carefully crafted menus provide some guidance. Servers then offer more tailored consultation. SC2.0 supplies both levels of direction. This may be less true in the context of pathways models. Instead, the selection is decided for them. Imagine a restaurant where dieticians decide your meals for you. Perhaps they would base these on your body type, fat levels or pallor.

Service pathways are predetermined, based on symptom cut-off scores. If your PHQ-9 score is above x, then you will receive this fortifying meal high in protein and rich with antioxidants (high-intensity programming). If it is less than x, you might receive a snack of fruit or nuts (low-intensity programming). To me, this is not much different from putting up a fence around the campus bowl. The approach curbs desire. In the context of mental healthcare seeking, it throttles motivation, or in the words of Michael Hoyt and Moshe Talmon, it fails to "capture the moment" of opportunity that presents when a help-seeker first reaches out (Hoyt & Talmon, 2014). There is an energy that drives all requests for mental health support. This is a rare, wonderful type of energy, especially given that a struggling person may not be firing on all cylinders.

Staging models are certainly well-intentioned. There is a clear and simple logic to them. Give more to people who appear to suffer more. Give less to those who suffer less. After all, the risk is higher with those who suffer more. Or is it? What do we know about the relationship between symptom severity and risk? How good are we at risk assessment? According to several meta-analyses on suicide screening and suicide prevention, we are not very good at all. There is no evidence showing either approach saves lives (Harrod, Goss, & DiGuiseppi, 2014; Zalsman et al., 2016). Instead, there are some indications that deficit-oriented screening assessments without much attention to support might be harmful (Klimes-Dougan, Klingbell, & Meller, 2013).

In the case of Lake, outlined above, a staging approach would have led straight to intensive therapy. At our counselling centre, this would mean seeing a senior psychologist with a high level of expertise and a high salary. Lake's care preference was for one-on-one regular support, but they were not interested in intensive psychotherapy. When asked to describe what worked previously, it became clear that they were looking only for support. A semester-long course of active listening is not a Step-7 intervention. Lake was not ready to be challenged. I could have spent weeks attempting to nudge Lake towards therapy readiness, but in our SC2.0 approach, we do the reverse. My task was to connect Lake with something they were ready for at that very moment. To guide Lake to an option that fits their readiness, not mine. A trainee fit the bill. This does preclude some nudging. I tried some. Lake was intrigued by the possibility of accepting a greater challenge, just not quite ready. Preference is very important, but it comes with conditions. Lake may have wanted an experienced clinician, and they could have had one, but that option depended on their willingness to engage in difficult work. With this condition made clear, Lake chose to see a trainee for supportive counselling.

5.3 What Should Guide the Adjustment of Care?

How and under what circumstances, should we provide guidance while still honouring preference? With respect to desire paths, some features of the natural and built environments will inevitably restrict choices. A person is not likely to climb a steep hill if it is easy to walk around it. Trees will have to be skirted, and movement through buildings is limited to entrances. Consider those road signs that flash your current speed. Placed strategically near busy crosswalks or school zones, they may prompt a driver to slow down. There are no instructions. It is just feedback. Other roadway design features, while even more subtle, may have more direct influence. Traffic-calming structures influence a driver's perception of safety. For example, a curb or sidewalk that juts out into the road leads most drivers to slow down because high speed on a narrow roadway feels uncomfortable. But again, it is a choice left to the driver. Given that preference, along with readiness and autonomy, are paramount in recovery models, could our mental health guidance tools somehow mirror these roadway features?

But first, let us consider more precisely what we need to measure in order to guide treatment choices. Decades of research should point us in the right direction, but as is often the case with research data, interpretations vary. Over the past 30 years, much discourse has contributed to "the great psychotherapy debate", a term coined by psychologist Bruce Wampold (Wampold & Imel, 2015). The debate involves two camps of researchers and clinicians: (1) those who believe diagnoses and specific techniques tied to these classifications are a key to good outcomes and (2) those who believe that common (or non-specific) factors, such as therapeutic alignment, context, modality, and uncontrollable situational variables determine outcomes. While these positions are not mutually exclusive, there remains a deep divide, particularly among researchers who influence policy and ultimately programming decisions.

According to Bruce Wampold, the debate has been won. The common factors are more important (see Table 5.1). Meta-analyses and studies applying multiple regression have consistently found that techniques and diagnoses account for less than 15% of outcome variability. Approximately 45% of the variance is due to unpredictable life circumstances like car accidents, an economic recession or natural disasters (Hubble, Duncan, & Hubble, 1997). The good news is that SC2.0 is well-positioned to respond even to the unpredictable extra-therapeutic events. But SC2.0 is especially attentive to the 40% of outcome variance attributable to the therapeutic context variables.

The debate raises questions about the nature of evidence. If diagnoses and techniques are not predictive of outcome, then how can we ensure treatments are informed by evidence? Some of the most vocal proponents of "evidence-based psychotherapies" insist that a very specific set of techniques such as cognitive behavioural therapy (CBT) merit gold-standard approval. This in itself is misleading, given that technique only accounts for 15% of outcome variance at best. Furthermore,

Table 5.1 Estimated variance accounted for by therapeutic factors

Source of therapeutic outcome	Portion of variance accounted for
Techniques and assessment	Less than 15%
Extra-therapeutic factors • Patient circumstances • Unpredictable events • Patient motivation	Approximately 40%
Therapeutic context • Therapeutic alignment or engagement • Accessibility of care (e.g. immediate or wait time) • Modality of care (in person, web, text) • Expectations	Approximately 45%

effect sizes in clinical trials of most types of psychotherapy are moderate or high with little variation. The gold standard stamp of approval for CBT simply cannot be justified. However, and it warrants repetition, specific factors, such as techniques are not independent of the much more impactful non-specific factors. It would be hard to develop a solid therapeutic alignment or generate hope (positive expectations) without offering a method of care. The point is that misleading claims of evidence should not dictate choice of treatment. What matters more is the fit for both therapist and client, along with tenacity to champion the choice itself with compassion, openness and flexibility.

SC2.0 endorses practice-based evidence over evidence-based treatments (see Table 5.2). Evidence-based treatments typically emphasize the importance of fidelity to a manualized protocol. Historically these were different for every diagnosis. The importance of diagnosis has decreased over the past decade. Psychologist David Barlow, who published several influential texts in the "Treatments That Work" series, each corresponding to a specific diagnosis, has since recanted. He now promotes the "transdiagnostic unified protocol" in recognition that patient distress regardless of diagnosis is all that matters in treatment planning. But SC2.0 moves even further from protocols. Instead of relying on clinical trial evidence for a specific treatment method, we simply monitor how a person's unique, chosen pathway affects their recovery and when recovery is stalled or deteriorates, guidance is offered to carve a new path.

5.4 Therapeutic Measurement

Systems designed for therapeutic measurement, also known as feedback-informed treatment (FIT), have been around for more than 20 years but are still not part of routine practice. One the one hand, this is surprising given solid research indicating that outcomes improve by up to 50% when used at every point of contact (Miller, Hubble, Chow, & Seidel, 2015). For those committed to FIT, most use one of two

Table 5.2 Evidence-based treatments versus practice-based evidence

Evidence-based treatments	Practice-based evidence
Evidence is derived from controlled randomized clinical trials	Evidence is derived from continuous therapeutic progress measurement
Specific factors/techniques are manualized	Treatment may be based more on common factors and/or may not be manualized
Fidelity to the manual is priority	Fidelity to the relationship is a priority; fail forward by adjusting techniques
Contextual factors may be considered a confound	Contextual factors are key therapeutic ingredients
Outcomes tend to focus on symptom reduction	Outcomes are more broadly defined
Favours techniques that can be clearly isolated and logically operationalized	Supports flexibility, wide range of techniques and integration

systems: the OQ-45 or the ORS/SRS. Both have good psychometric properties and have the capacity to alert clinicians when treatment is not progressing as expected. As the name implies, the OQ-45 contains 45 items most of which target a broad range of mental health symptoms or deficits.

The ORS/SRS, in contrast, is much shorter and not symptom-based. The ORS contains four broad recovery-oriented items each using a continuous scale. For example, with the first item, clients are asked to rate how they are doing "individually" by sliding a dot to the left (not doing well) or to the right (doing well). The other items capture interpersonal, social and overall functioning. It is a simple tool to administer and has non-verbal as well as telephone versions. The SRS is a complementary 4-item scale that targets alignment with the therapist. For example, the first item invites clients to rate the therapeutic "relationship" by moving the dot to the left towards "I did not feel heard, understood, and respected" or to the right towards "I felt heard, understood, and respected". The three remaining SRS items track clients' perception of alignment on "goals and topics", "approach or method" and "overall" satisfaction of the session. Although there are no symptom items, the ORS has been well validated against some of the best symptom rating scales.

A popular tool for post-secondary settings is the CCAPS (Counseling Center Assessment of Psychological Symptoms). It is quite like the OQ45 in length and its focus on symptoms. Given its wide use in college and university counselling centres, it is often used for benchmarking a centre's performance.

We used all three tools at Memorial University. The OQ45 and the CCAPS are longer instruments that take more time to administer. We also found them less conducive to collaborative step decision-making. Clients reported survey fatigue and counsellors did not find them helpful for giving continuous feedback or initiating conversations on treatment decisions. At a recent conference for Counselling Centre directors, I facilitated the Stepped Care Affinity Group meeting. There were about 100 directors in the room. When I polled the group to identify those using the CCAPS, the majority raised their hands. When I asked if anyone used it for every session (for which it was designed), no hands went up. The most common response was using it only at intake, followed by once every four sessions. This is not feedback-informed treatment. It is periodic outcome assessment, conducted too infrequently to inform nimble stepping decisions.

When we tried to use the ORS/SRS at our counselling centre, clinicians felt something was missing. Specifically, while they wished to move away from simply tracking deficits, they did not appear ready to let go of some monitoring in this area. Especially for an initial encounter, counsellors liked having some information on symptom patterns available on their desktops especially before greeting clients in the waiting area. We eventually landed on the BHM-20. While less well known, it does have reasonable psychometric properties and captures much of what is relevant to SC2.0 (Bryan et al., 2014). Specifically, it is brief—only 20 items and takes at most 90 seconds to complete. It includes separate symptom, wellness, functioning, readiness and therapeutic alignment scales. In contrast to most other outcome tools but in line with recovery principles, a high score on any BHM scale implies good health. Finally, the reporting functions are user-friendly especially for the purposes of reviewing alongside clients.

5.5 The Case of CK

A common myth associated with SC2.0 is that it oversimplifies therapy and as a result has little value for complex cases or severe and persistent mental illness. Nothing could be further from the truth. CK is a fictional client based on an amalgamation of case material from four clients with complex and severe illnesses (see Table 5.3). They all encountered SC2.0 and in one case, experienced care both prior to and following implementation. Identifying information has been disguised. The flexible nature of SC2.0 is revealed in the stops and starts and back and forth of CK's journey. The first section is a summary of case notes on file prior to the implementation of SC2.0. Her open-access walk-in presentation is denoted as a "Step 0" intervention. This entry point is marked with the open-access box in Fig. 1.2 in Chap. 1.

5.6 The Case of TD

Stepped care is also being implemented in community settings focused on treating operational stress injury. As with CK, the case of TD is based on an amalgamation of case material from several real clients at the clinic. This case was prepared by my colleague, Dr. Kyle Handley, who at the time of writing was lead psychologist at a large city police department in Canada. SC2.0 was adapted for use in the stress injury clinic. As indicated in Fig. 5.1, steps are based on the Road to Mental Readiness (R2MR) mental health continuum model developed by the Department of National Defense (Government of Canada, 2020). The journey is different for TD. Like many first responders, TD was concerned that formal treatment might require disclosure that could compromise his employment status. These are legitimate concerns. There are indeed policies requiring disclosure of diagnoses and treatment that could affect an officer's right to carry a badge or a firearm. Not surprisingly, TD preferred peer support and self-help options (see Table 5.4).

5.7 FIT for the Future: A Prototype

Currently, on the East Coast of Canada, we are working on a research project funded by the Canadian Institutes of Health Research (CIHR) to fully digitize SC2.0. One of the aims of the project is to develop a platform and portal to automate therapeutic measurement and ensure better access to these data for both help-seeker and

Table 5.3 CK's Stepped Care 2.0 journey

The case of CK—a student with complex PTSD	CK is a 24-year-old female graduate student seeking a Master's of Health and Humanities degree. She first came to the Student Wellness and Counselling Centre in her third year of her undergraduate studies for treatment of symptoms of anxiety and depression. The case notes for this previous therapy indicated that initially the focus was on symptom reduction and family of origin dynamics related the breakup of her parents' marriage (when she was 7 years old) as well as long-standing conflict with her mother. After some initial symptom management and interpersonal focus on family dynamics, CK disclosed that she had been sexually assaulted over a period of 4 months when she was 9 years old by the son of a visiting pastor in her small community where she was living at the time with her mother. CK eventually disclosed the abuse to her mother who responded, "That's just what boys and men are like" The case notes revealed that CK had not disclosed the assault to her father who she said still thought of her as his "little princess" who could do no wrong. CK was estranged from her father, who had remarried shortly after the divorce. CK said that her mother had actively discouraged her from making contact with her father who she argued was a "sexist and selfish man". CK described her mother as emotionally unstable and frequently angry. She admitted that she had a somewhat romanticized view of her father based on early childhood impressions. The previous therapist noted that although CK was quite forthcoming about "the bare facts of her life", she seemed distant and emotionally restricted during the sessions. CK admitted that she was unsure about the potential for therapy and that she struggled to let anyone help or get close to her. She indicated that she was not comfortable talking about the childhood abuse. She stopped therapy abruptly
STEP 0—Walk-in Consult	When CK returned 5 years later, the stepped care model had been implemented. CK completed the BHM-20 in the waiting room. At the walk-visit with me, CK said that she wanted to resume therapy because her father had been diagnosed with terminal cancer. Although she appeared calm in the session, her posture was stiff, and she reported having severe anxiety and panic attacks weekly. When I queried her about a preference for a male or female therapist, CK said that she finds it extremely difficult to open-up to new people but generally felt less anxious talking to males because they are more direct and trustworthy. CK's readiness for psychotherapy score was low. Although her suicide index scale score was in the severe range, CK said that she did not intend to kill herself, had never attempted or developed a plan. She reported having numerous protective factors which included her husband of 3 years, two very close friends and a passion for her studies. The new treatment model was explained and after a brief interview we developed a preliminary treatment plan to address her top priority—anxiety reduction. I demonstrated a simple technique for mindfully welcoming and "weathering" panic attacks and summarized the treatment plan on our behavioural prescription form. Included on the form was an invitation to contact me over the next few days via email should she wish to return or alter the plan
STEP 5—Therapist Assisted Online	Three weeks later, CK attended my walk-in again. She shared her decision to engage in some ongoing work. Given CK's low readiness and discomfort with face-to-face interaction, a low-intensity program plan was developed collaboratively. The program focused on developing anxiety coping skill sessions using online treatment modules and weekly 15-min face-to-face therapeutic coaching sessions. CK said that the shorter face-to-face sessions would feel less overwhelming. Session-by-session progress monitoring revealed increasing symptoms but a strengthening therapeutic alignment
STEP 7—Flexible Intensive Individual Therapy	As a result of the deteriorating symptoms, and in light of the strengthening alignment and readiness, care was stepped up to weekly face-to-face 50-min sessions. As the therapeutic alignment ratings gradually climbed, CK began revealing details of her troubled childhood, including the sexual abuse. We explored the impact that both the abuse and her mother's dismissive response had on her development. CK admitted that on the one hand, she learned to be tough and independent "on the outside", while inside she felt numb, and at times, like a "scared little girl". Despite the growing therapeutic bond, CK's symptoms continued to worsen as her father's health deteriorated

STEP 8—Specialist Consult	In consultation with her family physician, CK was referred for a one-time consult to our psychiatrist who diagnosed her with complex PTSD and recommended antidepressant treatment. After 6 weeks, symptoms stabilized but did not improve
STEP 7—Flexible intensive Individual Therapy	With the stabilization of CK'S symptoms, we began a course of prolonged exposure therapy which allowed some creative processing of the abuse experience and aftermath; however, she reported continued dissociative experiences that were easily triggered by news events or interpersonal conflict. Weekly monitoring using the BHM-20 indicated to both of us that therapy was not progressing. Furthermore, CK admitted that her interest and attention to her graduate studies were waning and that she was becoming emotionally dependent on the weekly therapy hour. We agreed that a shift in the treatment plan was needed
STEP 9—Acute Care, System Navigation & Advocacy (includes "Creative" Case Management—e.g., Peer led "Client Design Team")	With CK's interest in psychology and health, we decided that assigning her to our new "client design team" would allow her to connect with peers to research, consult on and adjust our stepped care service model to better meet the needs of students, including herself. Given her high depression scores, low energy and the emergence of some anhedonia, we recognized that the project would be challenging, requiring additional support. As such, while this referral involved stepping up to Step 9, weekly therapy at Step 7 continued. The work on the client design team provided her with opportunities to discover and apply strengths and capacities in a group setting by drawing on her lived experience. The occupational therapy type of support on the design team was high intensity. CK's contributions to the design team were well received and led to the development of a new second stage "living-room like" waiting area for anxious patients. On her own initiative, CK reduced therapy session frequency. Over time, she reported increased interest in her studies, including selection of a research topic related to mental health. Although her anxiety symptoms as measured by the BHM-20 remained high, her life functioning and well-being scale scores improved to a healthy range. CK said that her dissociative episodes and panic attacks were becoming rare and attributed to healthier distractions. She explained that she was now busier with activities she finds rewarding and meaningful. She said there is "less room for those old feelings now". CK continued with half hour, biweekly sessions which have focused increasingly on her graduate study and career interests. CK decided to end therapy and follow up only as required

Table 5.4 TD's Stepped Care 2.0 journey

The case of TD—A first responder with PTSD	TD is a police constable with 16 years on duty as a patrol officer. In the past 8 months, his supervisors have noticed a change in his behaviour while on duty, with several instances of being caught speeding in his cruiser, a sharp increase in his pay duty hours and two public complaints regarding his abrasive interactions with the community. Recently, TD was sent home after his supervisor smelled alcohol on his breath when he arrived for his night shift. TD was referred to his service's staff psychologist and though he was initially reluctant, he agreed to attend voluntarily
STEP 1—The Initial Consult	TD presented as highly guarded and defensive during the intake session, resisting efforts to explore his history aside from the documented behavioural concerns on the job and demonstrating a discomfort with questioning related to the emotional impact of these situations. Though he explicitly denied experiencing any suicidal ideation, he was evasive when his alcohol use was probed, insisting that his dismissal from his night shift was an overreaction and that it was only because he had a beer with dinner shortly before leaving for work. Noting his resistance, the staff psychologist explored TD's reaction to being referred for counselling. TD was adamant that he is "not crazy" and expressed his concern that both his recent behaviour on duty and his referral to counselling will erode the trust he has built with the fellow officers on his platoon and make him look "weak". Referencing the Mental Health Continuum, the staff psychologist suspected that TD was in the orange or "injured" category and offered an intervention appropriate to his level of need. Acknowledging TD's concerns, the staff psychologist recommended follow-up with a designated peer supporter on a separate platoon as a means of expanding his available coping resources and offering a perspective from a fellow officer with lived experience of work-related mental health concerns. TD agreed that he would be more comfortable speaking with a fellow officer at this stage and booked a follow-up with the staff psychologist to report back on his experience
STEP 4—Drop-in Peer Support/Chaplaincy	In his second session, TD reported that he had a positive meeting with his peer supporter, who shared his own history with PTSD and the warning signs he missed as his symptoms escalated. TD explained that he found the peer supporter's story mirrored his own in many ways, making note of how a slowly encroaching emotional numbness impacted his relationships at home and at work. He went on to reflect on several calls he has attended in his career that he now acknowledged contributed to the decline in his mental health, including one in which he was unable to resuscitate a 16-month-old who had fallen into a pool and drowned. Speaking with the peer supporter helped him understand why he would experience intense physical reactions when receiving calls for service related to children in danger, as well as the ways he attempted to dull his emotions by becoming withdrawn and increasing his alcohol use. After consulting the Mental Health Continuum, TD stated that he still feels as though he is in the orange category and recognized that he has more work to do to improve his psychological health
STEP 7—Intensive Individual Therapy with Psychologist	TD agreed to participate in a course of one-to-one individual therapy to help him "get back to the green" At the conclusion of TD's course of individual psychotherapy, another consultation session with the staff psychologist was set up to discuss his progress. TD was noticeably brighter and more engaged during the session, demonstrating greater insight into his stressors and available coping resources than seen in previous meetings. He reported significant reduction in his symptoms as a consequence of diligent work with his therapist on his cognitive processing treatment but endorsed ongoing issues with sleep that he attributed to both physical tension in his body and difficulty adjusting to the changing hours of his shifts. TD reviewed the Mental Health Continuum with the staff psychologist, and they agreed that he is likely in the yellow or "reacting" category at this time
STEP 3—Interactive Online Self-Help	With this in mind, the staff psychologist provided TD with online self-directed psychoeducational materials on sleep hygiene and progressive muscle relaxation to help improve his sleep quality. TD thanked the staff psychologist for the resources and stated at the conclusion of the session that his engagement with these mental health services has helped him to become more self-aware and capable of recognizing the connection between his experiences on patrol and his psychological health

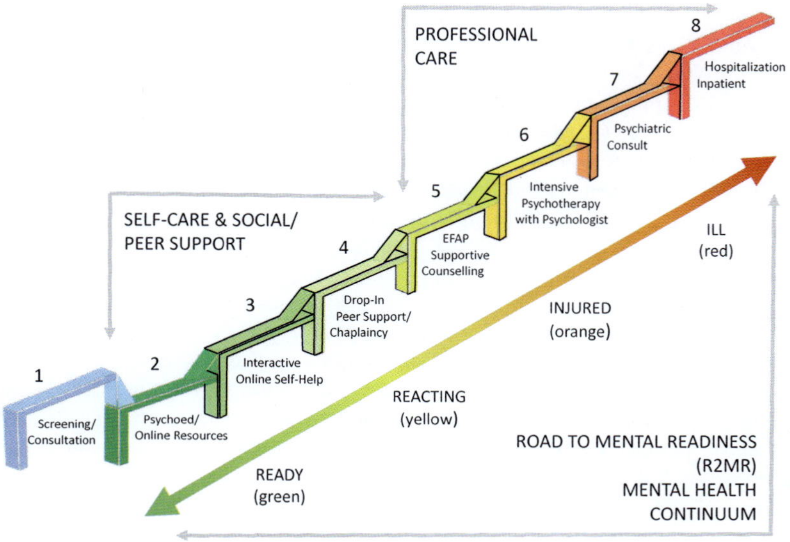

Fig. 5.1 Operational stress injury clinic version of Stepped Care 2.0

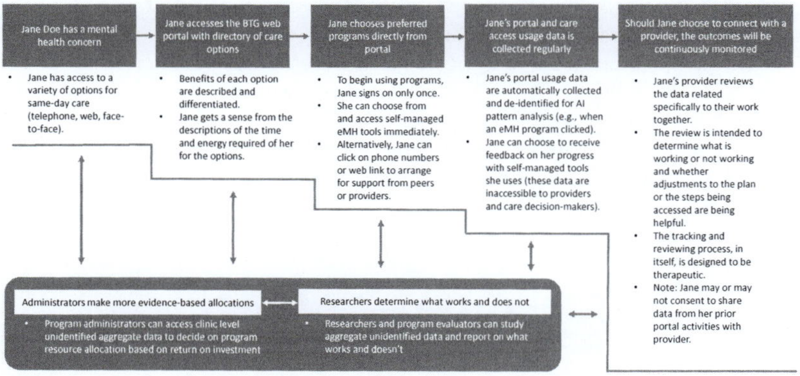

Fig. 5.2 Jane Doe's experience of proposed SC2.0 mental health platform

provider. At this point, we have created a storyboard that maps the journey we envision on the Newfoundland-based platform called Bridge the gApp. A client may decide to access tools online without being connected to a provider. The portal, of course, was not available when Amber (see Chap. 4) was looking for support, but if it had been, she may have taken a path like that of Jane Doe, illustrated below in Fig. 5.2.

The use of data should remain firmly in the control of the help-seeker. In the not-too-distant future, I envision a client-centric health system whereby the help-seeker is the only one with unfettered access to their own record. A provider might begin the session with, "Would you mind if I had a look at your health record?" The help-seeker would decide yes or no. If yes, with a few keystrokes on their phone, they could unlock the record enabling the provider to review. If no, the encounter would be treated as a one-at-a-time single session with no need to access the full record. The same principle would apply to the use of data collected through online care. The data belong to help-seekers. This is the default and applies until help-seekers consent to release. The release would require informed consent and specify the exact purpose for the release.

In the case of online program use without provider involvement, a pop-up greets Jane on her first web portal visit. The pop-up indicates that de-identified data will be collected and aggregated from Jane's interactions with the program. It would not be tied to her personal identity or shared with anyone unless she specifically requested this. It would not even be available for her to view unless she wanted to receive the feedback to guide her choices of programming within the portal. Finally, should Jane decide to work with a clinician, she would not need to release her data pertaining to the portal use, but could do so if she wished. The provider would indicate value in collecting data on their work together moving forward, but again this would be up to Jane.

Getting It Wrong to Get It Right

About 8 years ago, when stepped care was but a whisper in the back of my mind, I got a call from a woman named Susanne. She wanted care for her adult son who had been diagnosed with schizophrenia but was receiving only pharmacological treatment. I asked her how she thought I could help. She said she was told I operated a small private practice and that I had a reputation for working well with challenging cases. I said I wasn't confident that my type of therapy would help someone suffering from schizophrenia. She persisted, "There's lots of research now indicating that CBT and other therapies can help". I thought for a moment and said, tentatively, "Ok, go on". She continued, "Well the thing is, we've tried everything in the city. You are our last resort". My heart sank. Oh boy, I've heard this before, I thought to myself. "The other thing is, " Susanne continued, "He doesn't want to see you". Puzzled, almost hooked, I asked, "So what can be done?" She replied, "I will have to come in too". It was becoming slightly clearer. "Okay, so maybe a family therapy consult?" "No", she replied not missing a beat, "Just me and him". Reluctant but curious, I scheduled an appointment. Susanne and James arrived on time. After introductions, I asked James, what he thought would be helpful. He replied, "I don't think anything can help". Susanne interjected, "I think James needs some support. He has no one that he can talk to. Nobody wants to listen to him or his voices. Most professionals don't pay attention to the voices he hears. They just want to snuff them out with toxic drugs". I started to get nervous. I think Susanne noticed me stiffening. I was feeling out of my league. What do I do with this? Does she want me to suggest he stop taking meds? And what exactly does she want me to do with his voices? Meanwhile, James was quiet but looked increasingly bored, "I don't think this is going to help Mom. Can we leave now?" Susanne looked at me pleading. Her eyes said, "Do something Peter!" So, I pulled out the old standard and asked her what I should do. Susanne replied, "Do you know about the "Hearing Voices Movement". I said no. "It is a real thing," she continued, "There are people and families with lived experience and a growing number of professionals organizing in Europe and the United States to work more directly with the voices, the 'hallucinations' (with air quotes), to support them at times, to disagree with them at times, maybe by using CBT". James was getting more restless, "Let's go", he groaned. "I will email you some information on Hearing Voices", Susanne said hopefully, packing up her things. Reluctantly, I agreed to a follow-up. But the follow-up meeting did not go well. I was unconvinced. I tried half-heartedly to engage with some CBT exercises. Not surprisingly—he was no dummy—James could see me for what I was: unconvinced and uninvested. They left the second meeting disappointed and angry.

Fast forward 6 years. I am attending a regional stepped care implementation working group meeting by teleconference. There is a person with lived experience on the call. Her name is Susanne. I feel a vague yet uncomfortable sense that we may have crossed paths. But I don't make the connection. A few months later, she says something at another meeting that piques my interest. Under the Province's "Toward Recovery" strategy, specialists are not adapting their practices at all "in support of people with severe and persistent mental illness". Just before the meeting ended, I said I would like to learn more from her on this, perhaps we could have a separate call. Two months later, I receive a text from her. The text was sparse but blunt "You wanted to talk". It was then that it dawned on me, "Was this <u>that</u> Susanne?" We soon connected by phone. She had some suggestions about attending to the strengths of those with more serious conditions. Then there was a long pause. "We've met before, you know", she said. "I know", I replied now with full realization. "It didn't go well last time, did it?" I added. "No, it didn't". I thought for several seconds, then said, "I'm sorry. I didn't know back then. I didn't know anything about recovery".

And then 2 months ago, I am at a recovery conference in Montreal. It is a joint conference of the "Association québécoise pour la réadaptation psychosociale along with the "Hearing Voices Alliance". Who should I meet in the hall? Susanne! This time she gives me a big smile and says excitedly, "I have been talking about you. I didn't mention your name, but I have been telling everyone what you said". Smiling too, but with a puzzled frown, "Telling them what?" I asked. "I told them how important it was that you said, 'you said sorry and that you just didn't know'." My smile, a little bit shy now, widened, "I'm failing forward now". She leaned forward and gave me a heartfelt hug. "Too bad it took more than six years", I said sheepishly. After, I wondered what might have been different if SC2.0 had been in place earlier. And would therapeutic measurement have helped me to pivot quicker? Never mind, this is true co-design.

References

Bryan, C. J., Blount, T., Kanzler, K. A., Morrow, C. E., Corso, M. A., & Ray-Sannerud, B. (2014). Reliability and normative data for the Behavioral Health Measure (BHM) in primary care behavioral health settings. *Family, Systems, and Health, 32*(1), 89–100.

Government of Canada. (2020, January 12). *Road to mental readiness*. Retrieved from National Defence: https://strongproudready.ca/missionready/en/road-to-mental-readiness/

Harrod, C. S., Goss, C. W., & DiGuiseppi, C. (2014). Interventions for primary prevention of suicide in university and other post-secondary educational settings (Review). *Cochrane Database of Systematic Reviews*, (10), 1–88.

Hoyt, M. F., & Talmon, M. (2014). *Capturing the moment: Single session therapy and walk-in Services*. Crown House: Bethel, CT.

Hubble, M. A., Duncan, B. L., & Hubble, M. A. (1997). *Escape from Babel: Toward a unifying language for psychotherapy practice*. New York: Norton.

Klimes-Dougan, B., Klingbell, D. A., & Meller, S. J. (2013). The impact of universal suicide-prevention programs on the help-seeking attitudes and behaviors of youths. *Crisis, 34*(2), 82–97.

Miller, S. D., Hubble, M. A., Chow, D., & Seidel, J. (2015). Beyond measures and monitoring: Realizing the potential of feedback-informed treatment. *Psychotherapy, 52*(4), 449–457.

Wampold, B. E., & Imel, Z. E. (2015). *The great psychotherapy debate: The evidence for what makes psychotherapy work*. New York: Routledge.

Zalsman, G., Hawton, K., Wasserman, D., van Heeringen, K., Arensman, E., Sarchiapone, M., … Zohar, J. (2016). Suicide prevention strategies revisited: 10-year systematic review. *The Lancet Psychiatry, 3*(7), 646–659.

Chapter 6
Collaboration and Co-design

Contents

Client Design Team

"I just wanted somebody to talk to!" I could hear the exasperation in Melanie's voice even though it was an email she had sent to me over the weekend. Melanie was well known to our clinic. She had been given multiple diagnoses and was a frequent user of medical and mental health programming. She had a history of childhood trauma and strained relationships with her parents. She met the criteria for major depression and borderline personality disorder. Post-traumatic stress disorder was queried. She told us that she came to our university, in part, because it was 3000 km away from home. Her first contact with us was a "strong referral" from residence. She could come for counselling or be kicked out of residence for failing to follow the rules. Melanie used email frequently to connect with a variety of staff she had tried working with at our Centre. Boundary crossings were the norm for her. We set limits and one was that although she was free to send us messages, we would not reply to them except during office hours and only to suggest she make contact by phone or in-person when staff were available. She had signed a note promising not to send emails when in crisis and indicating her acceptance of the aforementioned conditions. On Monday morning, I replied to Melanie's weekend message. I said, come on in to see me, I am free for 20 minutes this afternoon. Melanie came in as requested and was angry from the outset, why wouldn't anyone see me? I came at 3:00 and was told the walk-in was full and no one was available to talk to me." I said, "Melanie, you know our system. There is no guarantee that a counsellor will be available later in the day. It is best to come early. If it is urgent, you know the crisis numbers in the community". "No, you aren't listening to me. I just needed someone,

P. Cornish, *Stepped Care 2.0: A Paradigm Shift in Mental Health*,
https://doi.org/10.1007/978-3-030-48055-4_6

anyone to talk to. It didn't have to be a counsellor". I was intrigued. "Who were you hoping to talk to?" "Anyone", she said, "Patty or Jen on the front desk, I don't know". I thought for a moment, or maybe a peer helper?

6.1 What about Boundaries?

Despite considerable distress, difficulty maintaining social relationships, chronic suicidal thinking, Melanie was actually very high functioning. It puzzled me at times. How could she be getting through her Pharmacy degree when her mood was chaotic and her relationships with staff in residence and our clinic were so volatile? Melanie had strengths. She had competencies. In addition to academic success, she had led in the development of a mental health advocacy alliance on campus. The group lobbied for improved mental health programming and later committed to the development of a peer support program. It was ironic that Melanie was asking for this kind of support. During our conversation, we agreed to two things: She would reach out to her peer advocacy group and I would investigate the possibility that our administrative staff be trained to provide support (a listening ear, perhaps in the quiet room). It turns out that two of our front desk staff, Patty and Jen, had the right skillset and temperament for this. In fact, both Patty and Jen were delighted with the opportunity to provide support to students in crisis. They had already had mental health first aid training and had naturally sound listening skills. Jen said to me in passing a few months later, that the invitation to provide such support in the quiet room was a turning point for her. She explained that the feelings of stress and lack of recognition she had been discussing with me for years had dissipated since she was offered this role. It was a meaningful role that complemented her clerical duties.

When I shared Melanie's story with colleagues eager to learn about our SC2.0 model, some asked about boundary crossings. "How do you handle ethical concerns associated with dual relationships with clients like Melanie who are known for their poor boundaries?" I typically give a two-part response: (1) ethical care does not prohibit boundary-crossing – after all, boundary crossings are inevitable. What is required is good boundary management and (2) I let go of the risk paradigm and believe in my clients' capacities despite their deficits.

6.2 Who Comes to the Table and When?

Post-colonial theory reminds us of the lasting impact of oppression. People with mental illnesses have suffered oppression perhaps more than any other group. They have long held the top spot of most marginalized and disenfranchised. The "cures" at times are the epitome of barbarism. The mental health recovery movement aims to redress this. But our steps in this direction are tentative. We are still walking on eggshells. I don't think any of us are ready for full reconciliation. We are not sure what this could look like or how to go about it. But we are making some strides.

This ambivalence is evident in my own approach to co-design. We hear from those with lived experience that they must be at the table at the very beginnings of any mental health reform efforts. But I am too impatient. I envision with some dread, the long circular conversations, a chaotic bubbling up of disparate ideas, grievances and no semblance of a cohesive plan. How can we bring bold transformation in the context of anarchy? With some guilt and worry that my need for control represents a form of neo-colonialism, I propose that we must create something before we take it to the masses for input. I convince myself that the consultations will be genuine, and that co-design will happen soon. But first, let me propose the idea. Let's start with something concrete and systematic. Let me show you the forest and the trees. If you wish, you could tear it down. But I am hoping it will inspire us all to work together to cultivate the new landscape.

We were thinking of this dialectic when planning our focus groups near the end of our first SC2.0 demonstration project in Newfoundland and Labrador. While piloting the questions among a few people with lived experience of mental illness, we discovered participants knew little about our project, stepped care, or e-mental health. They *could* tell us about their experiences with the mental health system in general, but would they know, or would we know if this feedback pertained to our work? Surely this is not a unique conundrum. We thought about how advertising campaigns are tested and refined before launch. Fly a trial balloon in front of a carefully selected, captive audience. We needed to fly a balloon, but we did not have one. What could it look like for SC2.0? Maybe we could draft up the elevator speech. But could we capture the complexity and the power we see in the model in a short speech? We needed a killer explainer video. So that's what we did. Now when we visit communities and invite stakeholders to help us build a model to fit their unique culture and circumstances, we start with the video. The idea is to inspire and then let the ideas stretch out while retaining connection to the core principles.

6.3 SC2.0 Distributive Design Cycle

Our design process starts from the centre and works outward. It is based on a principle we call *distributed co-design* (see Fig. 6.1). This means that co-design is distributed progressively outward starting with thought leaders and then incrementally incorporating broader input from experts and non-experts. The first step (at the centre in Fig. 6.1), is to assemble a small design leadership team comprised of clinicians and scientists who are grounded in recovery principles and theory as well as open and passionate about system transformation. This group is like a team of architects tasked with rethinking a build from the bottom-up. Like many architects, the initial designs may be somewhat fantastical with some inspiring yet ultimately unrealistic features. This becomes the ideal template for consideration at subsequent layers of the circle. We consult next at the inner circle with mental health clinicians

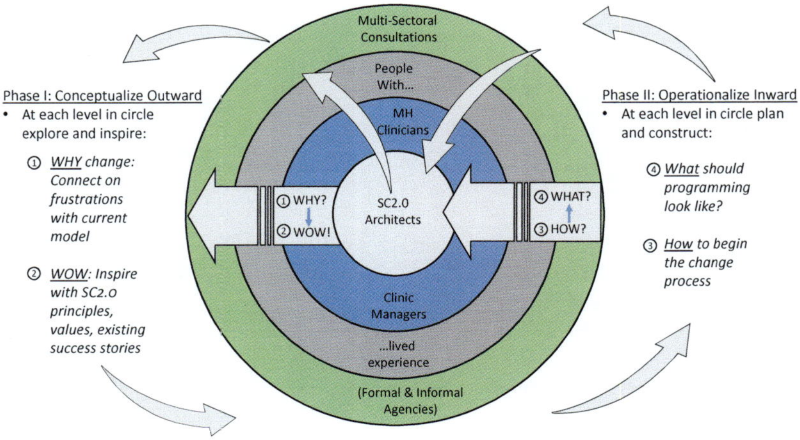

Fig. 6.1 SC2.0 Distributive Design Cycle (two-dimensional version)

and managers. We go here first because it is crucial to get manager and clinician buy-in and a sense of ownership of the system change process. Without some early feelings of ownership, clinicians might feel threatened especially if they think their roles and positions could at risk through restructuring. With clinician and manager buy-in and input, we take the modified template and move mid-circle, consulting with a broad representation of people with lived experience. At both the clinician and lived experience levels, we seek reactions to the model. What are the parts that inspire? What detracts from participants' own visions of mental health system reform? Can the proposed model be adapted or does it need to be torn down completely and rebuilt? Only after we have core stakeholder consensus (i.e. the first three circles) is it appropriate to expand consultation further through the larger community. These outer level consultations include stakeholders in the broader wellness ecosystem. Formal stakeholders at this level include thought leaders and decision-makers in primary, chronic, tertiary and acute care settings as well as representatives of public health, education, justice, social welfare agencies. Informal stakeholders include members of NGOs, and support groups like AA. While the initial concept prepared by the SC2.0 leads is considered first by clinicians and managers, then people with lived experience and last to external stakeholders, the development process then reverses so that the refined model can be operationalized moving in the opposite direction. We refer to this bi-directional process more formally as the "Distributive Design Cycle". It starts with initial ideas on *why* change and what might inspire (*wow*) us from the centre. These ideas are floated through internal, then external consultations. Then in reverse, we can consider *how* and *what* is needed through a narrowing needs assessment and environmental scan process. This reverse process gathers information from external stakeholders, which is then processed and refined by persons with lived experience. Then clinicians take this refined data and together with managers create feasible, adaptive programming that is well informed by all stakeholders. Further details on the Distributive Design Cycle (including the why-wow-how-what process noted in Fig. 6.1) are presented later in this chapter as well as in Chap. 7.

6.4 Interprofessional Collaboration

Client-centred and client-centric care cannot be achieved without breaking down silos. Without a formal process of interprofessional collaboration, care is fragmented. One professional ponders neurological chemistry, another contemplates social determinants of wellness and a third might consider lifestyle or cognitive processing. In a fragmented system, help-seekers are likely to be short-changed on several levels. They may get only the neurological perspective. Or maybe just wellness prescriptions. They might leave assuming it's just my faulty thinking. Even if the help seeker shops around and gets other perspectives, they miss out on the whole picture.

With all wearing blindfolds, no one sees the elephant. According to the ancient parable, they each "see" something through the sense of touch. They disagree on what is there and soon come to blows. Perhaps not unlike some interdisciplinary squabbles or turf wars. Pharmacists and pharmaceutical companies insist depression is a biochemical disease. No, say humanistic counsellors, it is a learned condition best resolved through discourse. You are both wrong says the sociologist. We need to adjust housing policies, redistribute wealth better and reform the justice system. But I wonder what the elephant experiences. Reputed to be quite intelligent, perhaps the elephant is insulted. "It's my leg, not a tree trunk. No, it's not a rope, it's my tail. Although I am big and strong, that's my stomach not a great wall!"

The blindfolds come off with interprofessional care. Instead of squabbling over turf, the group of observers communicate with each other to develop a holistic assessment. Perhaps most importantly, they invite the one being observed to weigh in, to express the preferred view or focus for attention. Without blindfolds, there still might be disagreement among observers. Why not let the elephant in the room decide. And why do professionals sometimes treat humans like they can't talk or that their preferences are not to be trusted?

Interprofessional collaboration is difficult to achieve. There are many barriers. First and foremost are the structural barriers. A licensed professional is by definition a protected guild defined in part by a defined scope of practice based on unique values, assumptions and perspectives. The various disciplines are stratified by power and authority, without much thought to rationale. Conflict and resentment are inevitable. Collaboration in this context is not very appealing.

What are the incentives for collaboration? Healthcare funders point to research suggesting outcomes are better and programming more efficient (Gilbody, Bower, Fletcher, Richards, & Sutton, 2006; Woltmann et al., 2012). But in order to shift practice, there needs to be incentive for professionals to stretch beyond their siloed practices. What's in it for professionals beyond a fear that others might encroach on their livelihood? How might collaboration enhance practice experiences of professionals? How can it allow them to improve their outcomes, or to decrease workload pressure, frustration and burnout?

One place to start is with identifying and exploring scope of practice. But without some sort of organizational structure this process might unravel. Before developing our SC2.0 model, I recall attempting interprofessional team building consultations that left participants more confused at the end. One of the topics that derailed the process centred on the question of who does counselling. The answer, of course, was that everyone did counselling—physicians, psychiatrists, psychologists, counsellors, nurses and social workers. Okay, so who does psychotherapy? "We all do". But what kind of psychotherapy do you do? "Mine is better than yours. Are you saying what I do is not helpful?" And so on.

Now when we consult on the topic of collaboration, we take a very different approach. Instead of beginning with who does what best, we take a similar approach to that of SC2.0 client care. We put aside our assumptions and preconceptions of who should do what and we simply ask about interests and preferences. But as with clients, we do not begin with a blank slate. Instead, we begin with the SC2.0 graphic. More specifically, we present it as a tool for scaffolding. Interventions, roles or competencies can be hung upon the various steps. They can decide where to climb on, whether they'll move up or down, and experiment with applying their tools and skills at any level. Where do they do their best work? Which work do they prefer? It is important that this kind of exploration be conducted as part of an interprofessional group exercise or workshop. The result will look different at every collaborative care site because the interests, motivations and skillsets will be different.

In some of these scope/scaffolding discussions, participants might want a bit more guidance. What sort of role differentiation has been successful? Are roles best distinguished according to professional discipline or is it better to consider competencies and interests? While not intended to be prescriptive, we have offered suggestions for both approaches as illustrated in Figs. 6.2 and 6.3.

6.5 Intersectoral Collaboration

One of the things that differentiates SC2.0 from other stepped care models is the deliberate effort made to expand the system to include and integrate supports from other sectors (beyond physical and mental health). These sectors include educators from kindergarten to post-secondary levels, public health practitioners, child welfare, the justice system, public housing and shelters, the clergy and Indigenous elders (see Fig. 6.4). Of growing importance are both formal and informal organizations of people with lived experience. Trained peer support is an example of the former. It usually requires training, certification and remuneration for services provided. Informal supports include naturally occurring support networks, self-help groups and organizations like AA.

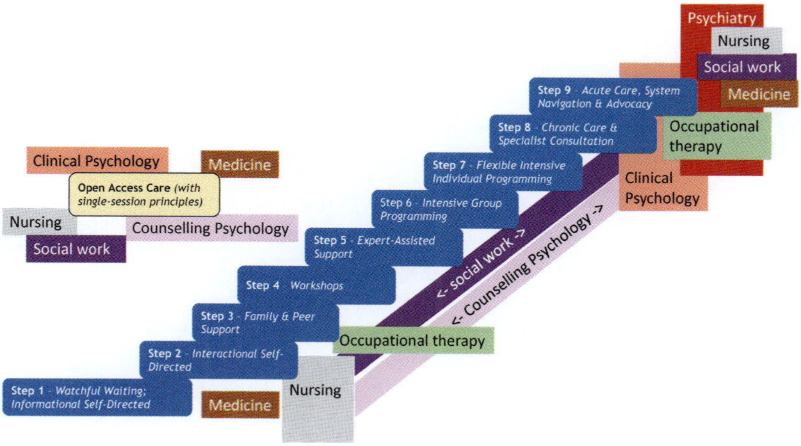

Fig. 6.2 SC2.0 scaffolding for disciplines

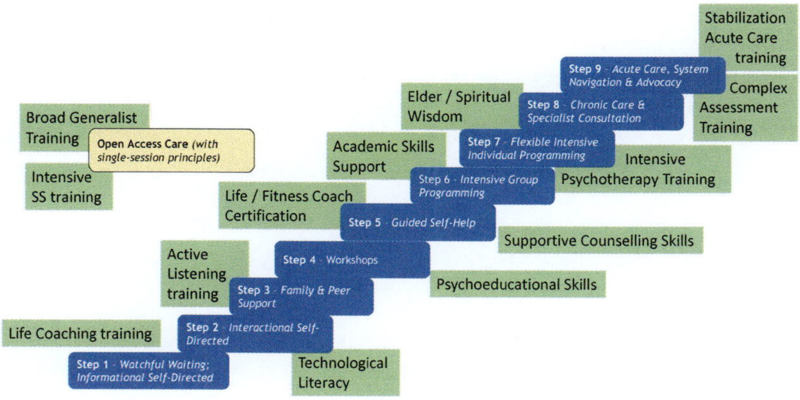

Fig. 6.3 SC2.0 scaffolding for competencies

In SC2.0 these non-clinic-based programs are considered population health-level programs since they are available to anyone whether healthy or ill. Indeed, part of what makes these intersectoral partners so powerful is that the mental health work is mainstreamed. It is of value to everyone. There is no sorting or stigma. A professor or a teacher is empowered to be a kind listener to all students whether ill or not. The same with clergy or Indigenous healers. A judge or a lawyer is supported to listen, communicate and show compassion to clients no matter who they are or what state they are in.

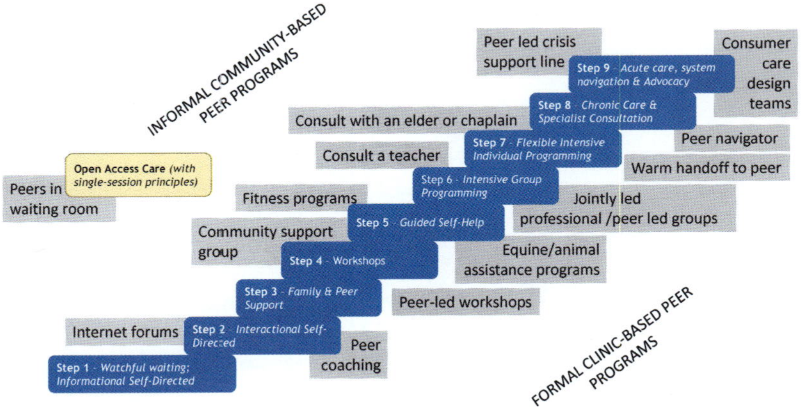

Fig. 6.4 SC2.0 scaffolding for intersectoral collaboration

Many professionals and non-professionals are interested in learning how to contribute to mental health. Who can help with this? As mental health practitioners develop more flexible and efficient ways of delivering care to their clients, they can pivot to provide consultation to external groups. There is synergy here. As more of this pivoting happens, intersectoral support will increase. As this external support increases, demand for clinical treatment will decrease. As a result, mental health resources expand.

6.6 Facilitating the Collaborative Aspiration

Client-centric care is empowering. To be empowered clients must be able to identify all the resources and the potential care providers available to them. They must know what to expect from the programs and what is expected of them in order to make choices. This information can only be clearly communicated if both programming and the providers involved from varied disciplines and sectors are organized and aligned in some fashion. This is a tall order especially given that not all professionals are fully committed to collaborative care, nor are there many structures in place to facilitate collaboration. SC2.0 provides a template for this structure. One way to operationalize the structure would be through the development of a therapeutic measurement platform. Such a platform, designed for ongoing progress tracking of recovery, could be embedded in electronic health record systems.

But there are a lot of "ifs" related to the social and structural challenges. First, this would only work if a common version of stepped care is widely adopted. Second, providers and mental health program decision-makers would need to agree upon and implement a common minimal dataset for progress tracking. Third, electronic health records would need to be configured and deployed across multiple disciplines and sectors. Fourth, collaboration is an idealistic concept. It is challenging for many understandable reasons beyond system development. Collaboration involves reaching across class and cultural divides built on inflexible societal power structures. Not only does client-centric care shift the power to individuals seeking care, it also requires some flattening of the medical hierarchy around with most healthcare is organized. Finally, conflict is inevitable in teamwork and needs to be attended to with care and flexibility. As such, supportive malleable structures like the SC2.0 model, with its underlying recovery principles, its commitment to co-design and its fail forward, trial-and-error philosophy, can provide a vehicle for working towards the collaborative ideal.

6.7 The Curse of Knowledge

My first attempt at writing Chaps. 6 and 7 fell flat. As I re-read this chapter, at least up to this point, it seems a bit dull. The descriptions on design processes are dry and overly technical. The variations of SC2.0 adapted and implemented by others described in my first draft of Chap. 7 seem dull and uninspiring. I recall feeling deflated and stuck with my writing. When I write, I typically start at the beginning and work my way to the end. These are crucial chapters. They must nail it. Chap. 7 is the last chapter of real substance; then Chap. 8 brings it home and links to the other two books in the planned series. Chap. 7, the penultimate chapter could not be a sleeper.

I suppose I did what anyone would do when blocked; anything except the task in front of me. Like many, one of my favourite distractions involves losing myself in social media. As an introvert though, all things social for me must have a purpose. It is perhaps not surprising that my medium of choice is *LinkedIn* where my connections are social but grounded in professional identity. As my posts on SC2.0 accumulated, my connections to others with a rebellious mindset expanded. I have been inspired by many a *LinkedIn* post. But with this case of writer's block, it was a message from Facebook that broke me free.

Recall Susanne from the closing in Chap. 6? The Facebook Messenger alert had lingered on my phone for about 4 days. I do not receive many of these and assumed it had something to do with a viral cat or cute toddler video. I didn't know who it was from. Because I had read all the news, exhausted my LinkedIn feed, was bored with my mystery novel, and tired of the endless mini crosswords on my phone, I ventured to Facebook—always a last resort for me. The message was from Susanne. It read simply, "You may like this". It included a link to an episode of NPR's Hidden Brain You 2.0 series. The title of the episode was *You 2.0: Rebel with a Cause* (Gino, 2018).

She had me with "You 2.0", but the rebel idea piqued my curiosity. It turns out, this was just what I needed. The episode spoke directly to me—a rebel in the field of clinical psychology. Host Shankar Vedantam was interviewing Harvard's Francesca Gino, a professor of Business Administration, who, among other things, studies non-conformists. The interview focused on "rebel talent" people who defy the status quo and create breakthroughs. She talked about Captain Sully. Unlike most leaders in emergency situations who typically narrow their focus and default to protocols, Sully decided to land in the Hudson River. He was clearly breaking the rules. What was it about Captain Sully, Gino wondered, that led to success? It wasn't because he had a lot of experience, which of course he did. Gino suggests that it was because he had overcome "the curse of knowledge". Often experts become set in their ways and impervious to new ideas. Sully, she argues, was a constructive rule breaker. He had what she calls "positive deviance". He had enough good judgement to know which rules must be followed and which could be broken. This requires tremendous risk-taking balanced with good judgement. Sounds like an oxymoron. It is probably quite rare. If risk-taking leaders do not have good judgement, both tact and empathy, or a willingness to express vulnerability, no one will follow them. Without this emotional intelligence and sensitivity, they would probably be considered arrogant and reckless.

So why was I stuck writing these two final chapters? The answer, thanks to Susanne, Francesca and Captain Sully: my writing had slipped into expert mode. The first draft of Chap. 6 was too technical and dry. It described stages, processes and recited facts. In Chap. 7, through my effort to anonymize the experiences of adaptation at various sites, the stories lost vitality. What was missing was my own vitality. The rebel that I am and my desire to throw myself completely into the tension between expertise and experimentation. I forgot to start with why. I did not ask why I was stuck until something new jolted me out of my expert mode and back into my rebel mode.

6.8 Rushing to Solutions

Transforming how we provide mental health services is, of course, difficult. Just as help-seekers are often not ready to make difficult lifestyle changes or fully participate in programs offered to them, care providers, administrators and decision-makers will approach change with caution. As leadership guru Simon Sinek suggests, it is important to begin with the *why*. Why change? What are the problems or needs that will be resolved with a change (Sinek, 2009)?

Many, including me, too often start with the *what*. I did just that at Memorial University about a decade ago. "I've got this great idea—this thing called stepped care. This is what it is", I began. I described it to my staff and after quickly answering a few tentative questions, I said, "Let's do it". Some staff said, "I'm not sure how to do this", or asked rhetorically, "Surely stepped care can't be used to organize everything we do?" I responded, "Oh really? Give me an example of something that won't fit?" Uncomfortable silence followed. I thought the question resolved and moved back to the what. Because the ideas I was talking about (this was the what), had piqued the interest of many colleagues across the country, I was encouraged to stay with the what. I was invited to deliver keynote speeches, to offer training, to consult. I spent a lot of time taking about ever more complex ideas which somehow retained their allure. Outsiders loved this. They loved the *what.* Organizations applied the ideas with some success and more interest was garnered. The ideas were connecting with needs of decision-makers and administrators even if they were not spelled out all that clearly. The needs included addressing long wait-lists and finding sustainable ways to manage risk. And the changes were received well by help-seekers, who noticed access to care improving.

But the "*why*" was not all that apparent to many practitioners. "Why should we change our practices? The training we have had, the research that we have studied, and our professional guidelines all say that what we are doing is appropriate. Why should we try something new that has not stood the test of time? And why should we do less assessment? What if we miss something? And, even worse, why should we shorten sessions? That will result in rushing clients and, ultimately, poorer quality service. What we really need is to hire more staff. We hear all the time that there are shortages of mental health professionals. The real solution is not change but increasing our investment in mental health to a level of parity with physical health. Problem solved".

In our consultations on implementation we soon learned that some vocal practitioners were not convinced that the model was a step in the right direction. Initially we simply chalked it up to the idea that "change is hard". That was what I did. Some of my staff just didn't have the right stuff, I thought with condescension. Or they weren't ready yet. They needed more nudging. Or I just needed to be patient. They will eventually see the light. This is like labelling as "resistant" all help-seekers who do not want the treatment you are offering, when it just might not be the right fit, or maybe the rationale for the approach had not been explained properly. How can we expect someone to embark on a challenging journey if we have not worked through to *why*? Like when we try preparing clients for treatment, the *why* must be relevant to them first and foremost. In the case of SC2.0, the *why* was reasonably clear and relevant to administrators and to clients, but not to many providers.

While SC2.0 was born at Memorial University and we improved efficiency, capacity and outcomes, the implementation faltered after about 5 years. My predecessor, a seasoned clinician and former director who was a gifted mentor to trainees and new hires had just retired. With his existential-humanistic principles and Socratic style, he had been the wise sage. While I had been urging transformation at breakneck speed, he calmed the waters, was the gentle voice of reason, reassuring all that the changes I was introducing were sensible. Several faculty members more retired. These staff were replaced with contractual hires. There was no job security. Either I hadn't noticed the rising anxiety and the muted signs of reluctance expressed by the new cohort or I did not want to acknowledge them. I had been buoyed by the enthusiasm my international director colleagues were showering on me at conferences for the bold new approach we had taken. But really, it was the new approach *I* had taken.

I recall a conversation I had several years ago with a colleague at the Association of University and College Counselling Centre Directors conference. Over a few gin and tonics, we were musing about leadership styles and asked ourselves what kind of leaders we were. I said that I thought my colleague was an "affiliative" leader because she focused on the emotional needs versus work demands of the staff. She creates harmony and builds emotional bonds. The motto is "people come first". While this certainly did capture the essence of her personality, she said, "Like you, Peter, I am visionary leader". Visionary leaders mobilize people towards a vision. The motto is "come with me". I agreed. That certainly was my style. But I said that I was not convinced this was hers. She replied, "True, I'm not really a 'come with me' person—I'm just going. I don't care if anyone follows!" I laughed. But inwardly, this puzzled me. I wasn't sure why, but I felt a little uneasy. While she is undoubtedly a bold, independent person who despises authority and even admits to being a conspiracy theorist, she is one of the most nurturing people I know. But the mischaracterization of her, it turns out, was not what troubled me. In hindsight, I learned that my discomfort was really about my own leadership, not hers. I was the real "I'm going" person. I had been the leader who failed to nurture the change in my own department. I went too quickly and expected people to follow blindly. I expected them to be as excited as some of my director colleagues, who numbering in the hundreds by this time, had been inviting me to visit their campuses and spread the magic of SC2.0. I had left my own staff behind. I realized that I could not reverse course. I was not an *affiliative* leader. My department is an academic unit, and I had led for three consecutive 5-year terms. Such a long tenure is unusual for academic leadership. A sabbatical was long overdue. Luckily, my successor, serving as Interim Director, *is* a nurturer. After a pause and a few steps back to recalibrate, the SC2.0 model is being adapted. I am confident that the model will continue to evolve at Memorial University as SC2.0 should.

6.9 Starting with Why

With lessons learned, our small SC2.0 consulting social enterprise (i.e. Cornish & Associates Stepped Care Solutions Ltd.) is now investing more effort in deliberate change management strategies informed by implementation science. We developed this process to ensure the right balance of leading with and focusing on bold ideas while nurturing collaboration, co-design and stakeholder buy-in. In order to cultivate interest in transformation, consultation must initially attend closely and persistently to the question "why" change. We have applied Sinek's "Why first" strategy to our Distributive Design Cycle introduced earlier in the chapter.

We start our work with institutional clients by helping them form a small SC2.0 leadership design team. This team moves gradually outward, consulting with staff, persons with lived experience and finally external stakeholders. As we move outward, we ask *why* change might be helpful and then, with reasons identified, we cultivate inspiring ideas. With real problems identified that are relevant to the audience at each level of consultation, they become primed to be *wow*ed! The process then reverses, gradually returning to the centre, bringing ideas of *how* and *what* will be implemented, first from external stakeholders, then people with lived experience and finally from staff. With the distributive design cycle completed, the leadership team has a solid, well-supported mandate to implement changes.

Initially, most interest in SC2.0 came from directors of college and university counselling centres who had seen me talk about it at conferences. I had successfully sold the *why* at these conferences and they were *wow*ed. Can you come and do the same with my staff? "Sure", I said, "I would be delighted". Over time, as I visited more and more centres, a method for why and wow emerged. It is an adaptation of a standard SWOT analysis, which I call "NOW. WOW! HOW?" (see Fig. 6.5). As a consulting team, we try to leave the *what* alone. "What" the model will be at the site evolves after we leave. The "why change" question is addressed through the first part of exercise which I call "NOW". In this exercise both clinicians and managers are invited to list first all the things that they are doing well, the things both they and their clients treasure, things they are proud of (indicated by NOW(+) in Fig. 6.5). These are programs and practices to be celebrated and preserved. Then they focus on the things that they are currently doing that are not working (indicated as NOW(−) in Fig. 6.5). These are frustrating, ineffective or both. These are things that they would like to eliminate if possible. Once this is done, participants are encouraged to shift to "blue sky" *wow* thinking. If you could do more of the things that you value, if you could change anything, imagine what it would look like. How would you feel delivering the adapted or SCALED-UP programs and what impact would they make? Were there things in my presentation at the beginning of the day on innovations achieved elsewhere that piqued your interest? Finally, the last phase of the exercise shifts to focus on the first steps in their program transformation process—the "how" of design. We only take a few tentative strides with *how* at this early stage. We have found that clinicians and managers are hesitant to move far with *how* without some further reflection and consultation with other local stakeholders.

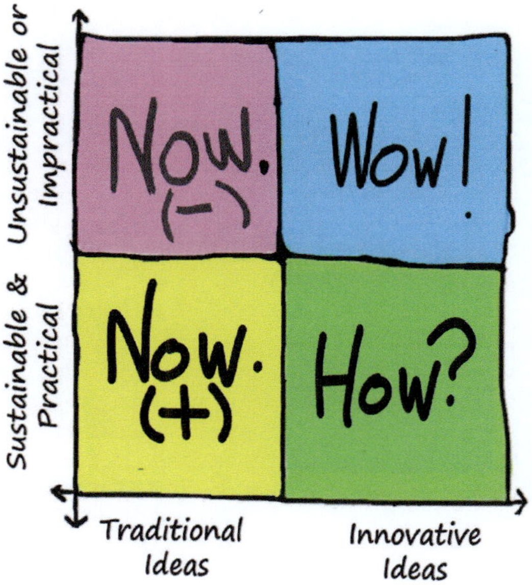

Fig. 6.5 Now, wow, how SWOT exercise

When we first started consulting, we worked only with site managers and their clinicians. The work centred mainly on the modified SWOT process described above. Since then we have discovered the power and potential of extending the design process outward to other stakeholders. Our Distributive Design Cycle incorporates and expands on the "now, wow, how" process.

After some training, reflection and follow-up discussion with site leads and clinicians, the next step is to engage with persons with lived experience. Some implementation experts suggest that persons with lived experience should be involved at the beginning and that any delay reflects an outdated paternalistic process. We disagree. Given that there is much higher anxiety about the changes among clinicians, it would be unethical to involve persons with lived experience at the beginning. To do so would be akin to a psychologically impaired clinician treating a client. In order for consultation to be productive, professionals and managers in authority roles need to get their house in order before working with either persons with lived experience or external stakeholders.

The distributive design cycle method is illustrated in more detail in Fig. 6.6. Consultation broadens in stages as we move up the spiral, beginning with site staff, then persons with lived experience and finally with external stakeholders. At each stage the issues are identified (WHY change), the ideas bloom and propagate (WOW possibilities), and the themes expand, evolving through the widening consultation

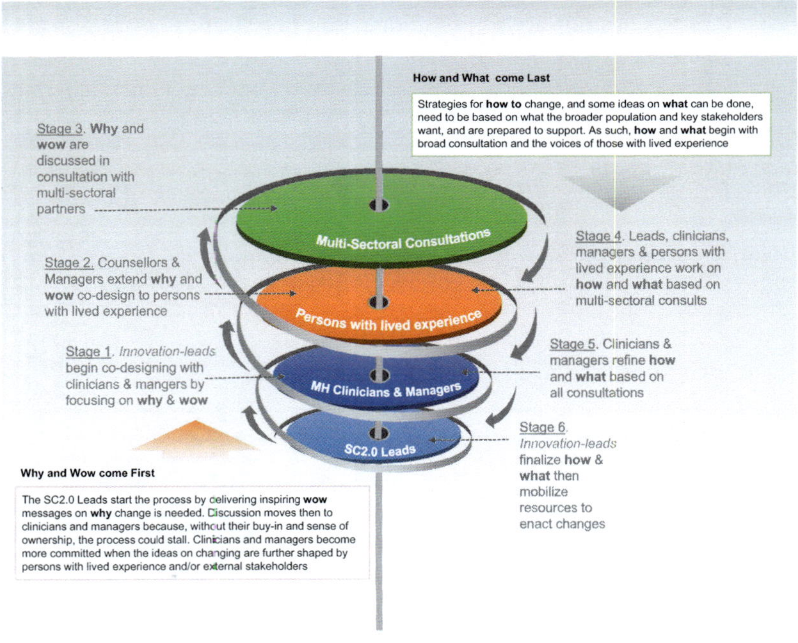

Fig. 6.6 SC2.0 Distributive design cycle (3-dimensional version)

process. Then moving from the top of the spiral back down, community-wide healing resources (broadly defined) are identified and configured (HOW do we implement) within the evolving SC2.0 template, integrated with more specialized informal and formal programs until the continuum of care can be clearly defined and implemented (WHAT). This process will become clearer in the next chapter, where it is applied in detail to a fictionalized case study based on an amalgamation of our experiences with institutions in both Canada and the United States.

Letting it Go

I came up with the name "Client Design Team" for a group of students who expressed interest in shifting how we provided care at Memorial University. I was supervising a graduate student, Brad, who was interested in developing peer support programming on campus. For at least 5 years, a mental health advocacy group called MUN Minds, had been funded by the undergraduate student union to support people with lived experience to advocate for improved programming. The group held fundraisers and awareness events and sometimes lobbied the University to do more to help students struggling with mental health issues. Recently the group indicated a desire to form a peer support network and asked Student Wellness and Counselling Centre staff to provide training. We did so. A collaboration began that preserved the group's autonomy. We trained students in mental health first aid, including active listening skills but we did not supervise their work. Instead, we made ourselves available for consultation, but only when requested by them. Brad helped with both the training and the consultation. He also mentioned to them our idea of forming a client design team. There were several members of MUN Minds who were also current clients. A few volunteered to join. Two counsellors also recommended the Design Team to their clients. TK (first introduced in Chap. 5) was one of them. They worked for about 8 months, reviewing de-identified client satisfaction data and learning about stepped care theory and research. Based on this work, along with their own lived experience, they wrote a report recommending adjustments to SC2.0. With Brad's guidance, they knew that the recommendations would have to be well-researched and feasible. They made a number of good recommendations that we implemented (e.g. plants in the waiting room, decreasing noise in the waiting room, a secondary quiet waiting area that also had more comfortable chairs and video games, the acquisition of a smart phone-based self-check-in system). But the recommendation that most surprised me was a name change for the Design Team. They did not like "Client Design Team". Instead, they wanted to call it "Students for Stepped Care". "That's not right", I thought. "You were once an advocacy group. You are disruptors and now we have co-opted you!" As with any true collaboration and client-centric system, Ironically, in this case, I had to let go of my "students-as-disruptors" vision.

References

Gilbody, S., Bower, P., Fletcher, J., Richards, D., & Sutton, A. J. (2006). Collaborative care for depression: a cumulative meta-analysis and review of longer-term outcomes. *JAMA Internal Medicine, 166*(21), 2314–2321.

Gino, F. (2018, July 23). *You 2.0: Rebel with a Cause*. (S. Vedantam, Interviewer) NPR. Retrieved November 30, 2019, from https://www.npr.org/2018/07/23/631524581/you-2-0-rebel-with-a-cause.

Sinek, S. (2009). *Start with why: How great leaders inspire everyone to take action*. London: Penguin.

Woltmann, E., Grogan-Kaylor, A., Perron, B., Georges, H., Kilbourne, A. H., & Bauer, M. S. (2012). Comparative effectiveness of collaborative chronic care models for mental health conditions across primary, specialty, and behavioral health care settings: Systematic review and meta-analysis. *American Journal of Psychiatry, 169*(8), 790–804.

Chapter 7
Adapting for Unique Settings

Contents

Why Change

"But isn't stepped care meant for clinics with inadequate resources?" A head-hunter for an Ivy League school expressed interest in my candidacy for Director of an integrated wellness and counselling centre. "With a multi-billion-dollar endowment, this school is not afraid to chart bold paths through innovation. Your approach might be just what they are looking for". I was impressed. My ego inflated. An Ivey League school might be interested in me? Not so, though, in the end. While the head-hunter was intrigued, she could not sway the committee. "We have lots of resources. We don't need stepped care", the Committee Chair reportedly said to the head-hunter. I had originally assumed as much. It had started as a model for an impoverished, remote Canadian province and our own under-resourced university counselling centre. But ever since I gave that 10-minute conference presentation in Chicago in 2015, I have been inundated with requests for consultation on our model from some of the unlikeliest places. One of the first is known by many as Canada's "Ivey league" leader. Initially, I had been invited to co-lead an administrative review of their mental health programming. I mentioned my work on stepped care during that visit and was invited back to present the model. At the time, this university had about 50 clinicians for 40,000 students. It has since increased the number of staff dramatically. Somehow, they still struggled with a long waitlist. They had an abundance of resources. The students were unhappy. The staff were unhappy.

P. Cornish, *Stepped Care 2.0: A Paradigm Shift in Mental Health*,
https://doi.org/10.1007/978-3-030-48055-4_7

Change was necessary. While the change process was complex and not without storming and controversy, the model was adapted to the unique culture of the institution and its commitment to be the best of the best.

7.1 Adaptation Stories and Processes

Our small consulting team, Cornish & Associates Stepped Care Solutions Ltd., has worked with over 100 colleges and universities across North America who have expressed interest in SC2.0. Recently, Provincial and Territorial Governments in Canada have contracted with us to introduce the model more broadly through the country's publicly funded healthcare system. A core feature of SC2.0 is its flexibility and adaptability. Some have remarked that it is more of a recovery care design process than a treatment model. It is certainly not a manualized program. In keeping with the principles of distributed co-design, it looks different in every location. The case study presented below describes co-design stories across all six stages of the implementation cycle. These have been drawn from experiences on our own campus and work we have done with a variety of institutions in both Canada and the United States. Many details have been changed to preserve anonymity.

7.2 Case Study: Large Mid-Western Public University

One of the first institutions we worked with is well known for its highly competitive admission standards and has solid reputation globally. Over the years this university had invested more in mental health than comparable institutions but the concerns about access had been raised by students. Was there duplication, were there inefficiencies, could we do better? A senior administrator asked me to serve on an external administrative review panel. We visited the campus and met with a variety of stakeholders internal and external to the department. We discovered about midway through the first day of consultations that representation from one key department responsible for addressing a large proportion of mental health programming was missing. We were surprised initially and then discovered that relationships between three student wellness service departments were strained. With a little initial resistance, we managed to arrange meetings with all parties.

At the end of the first day, during a break, I described our stepped care model to my fellow administrative review panellists. They were intrigued expressing interest in learning more. I said, maybe we could meet after our consultations are finished and I could share with both of you a presentation I delivered elsewhere. We asked one of the senior members of the department under review if we could get access to a room where I would have AV technology to present on my new model. Of course, the answer was yes. But, curious, this administrator asked if others would be welcome. We discussed privately as a panel and agreed to open it up to others. Four representatives of two of the three wellness departments attended. It was hard to read the interest of participants. The atmosphere in the room was somewhat guarded. Within a month our report was delivered. Among the recommendations, we suggested some steps be taken to improve collaboration among the units.

7.2.1 Stage 1: Initial Consultation—Getting to Why and Wow

I thought that was the end of my work with the University. However, about 1 year later, I was invited to present on the stepped care model to all clinical and administrative staff in the three wellness departments. I worked in advance with leaders of two wellness departments (the only two who were intrigued), to plan the agenda. The leadership teams of the two departments sat at the same table as me near the front of the room. I thought this was a good sign; the leaders were in this together. Collaboration was happening. There was both excitement and apprehension throughout the day of the workshop. Many were intrigued, however, a handful of very vocal critics held sway. These clinicians, some from each department were sceptical. Their questions at times bordered on hostility. It was, it turned out, the beginning of a period of significant storming.

Some of the clinicians filed grievances with their union. Others consulted with their professional organizations. SC2.0 was considered a potential threat to their professional autonomy, ethical practices and even their livelihoods. The model was perceived as prescriptive – mandating low-intensity, low-quality programming, some of which they feared would be facilitated by other professions, paraprofessionals or peer supporters.

I soon discovered that all was not well between two of the three leadership teams. One leader expressed serious concerns about SC2.0 and dropped out of the consultation process with us. Another leader, while not hostile to the SC2.0 model, did not see it as relevant at the time. Her department was not slated for amalgamation like the other two. The third leader continued to work with us, convinced that stepped care held promise. Despite the internal conflict, the University administration decided to go ahead with adapting the model. They invited me to visit again, this time to work with a smaller design team. The group on this team were enthusiastic and committed. This group knew *why* they were working on transformation and were *wowed* by SC2.0. However, one of the two departments had completely disengaged. The *why* did not seem clear to them. As such, collaboration between the units deteriorated. The one department that decided to go it alone received some institutional support. Lower intensity programs were launched including e-mental health tools and a rapid access system. The departmental leadership seemed pleased and I was too, but the transformation process was on shaky ground.

Our SC2.0 consulting team offered to help resolve some of the conflict between leaders of the two separate units that were to be merged at a future date. The unit that was more engaged with us was comprised of counsellors, psychologists and social workers. They identified as non-medical. The disengaged unit was more medically oriented; the mental health counsellors worked alongside health clinic staff, including physicians, psychiatrists, nurses and nurse practitioners. I was surprised initially that the medically oriented unit was not as interested in the model. Stepped care was initially developed for medical settings to improve coordination and transfer of care between primary care physicians and psychiatrists. But the drive for change had historically come from primary care practitioners who were frustrated with challenges accessing psychiatric care or consultation for their patients. At this University, psychiatrists were the majority among the staff of physicians, nurses, and nurse practitioners. The unit was led by a psychiatrist. All the staff psychiatrists worked fee-for-service which was covered by students' insurance. It was a private practice model of care. They did not receive benefits from the University and their allegiance was to their patients rather than the institution.

First, we met with the leaders separately to gauge their interest in mediation. They agreed only if the sessions would be structured according to an agenda developed in advance with their input. Over the course of 5 months, we met four times via web conference with the two leaders. An agenda was developed collaboratively prior to the first meeting and notes were "flip-charted" using the screen share feature. We carried forward the same agenda across all meetings, adjusting as we went along. Common goals were identified which include developing recommendations for:

(a) The relationship between the two leaders.
(b) More consistent revenue structures.
(c) Campus-wide consultations on mental health service reform and possible restructuring.
(d) How they envisioned their roles adapting through restructuring.
(e) Full implementation of an adapted version of SC2.0.

While the relationship between the two leaders had been strained, we got a sense that they liked each other. They recognized how their different styles were complementary. One was thoughtful and cautious, whereas the other was passionate and eager to act. Early on we also named 'the elephant in the room"—one of them might be vulnerable. Was one of their positions at risk with restructuring? We agreed after some discussion that it would be useful to explore the kinds of roles they envisioned with restructuring. It turned out that the administration was not in a rush to complete restructuring. Instead, they were interested in what both leaders would recommend following campus-wide consultations that had begun prior to our first contact with them. The University had a reputation for consulting widely and repeatedly on many issues. The focus of the consultation was vague. It was intended to gather all and any input on mental health experiences and ideas. After 5 months of consultation, and support from our team, the two leaders completed their report. It recommended a flatter organizational structure with a variety of adjacent lead roles. To facilitate development of the new care model (yet to be designed), the following lead roles were adopted: Healthy Campus Lead, Primary Care Lead, Mental Health Lead, Collaborative Lead and Stepped Care Lead. The report also recommended that the merger would ensure that all staff would be funded by a blend of insurance and operating revenue and that all would be eligible for benefits. The new money and matching central funds would allow for this.

7.2.2 *Stage 2: Public Relations Crisis—People with Lived Experience Lash Out*

In hindsight we had attempted to move too quickly to solutions. We had only gotten to the first step in the distributive design cycle—working at the inner circle with leaders. While we had made strides with the internal leadership team, we had underestimated conflict among staff. We thought we had solved some problems to their satisfaction. Low-intensity programming, including e-mental health tools, was helping to curb student demand already. Aligning revenue streams would bring clinical staff on board. And flatter leadership roles would ensure meaningful roles or existing leaders following restructuring. But the buy-in was not there. The two leaders had heard a number of complaints, but collectively we assumed we already had answers: low-intensity programming and stepped care. Yes, consultation had happened. Broad input had been obtained. But not true co-design. While all stakeholders agreed that demand for care had been exceeding supply, there was no shared perspective on why this was the case. Disregarding Sinek's appeal to always with "why" (Sinek, 2009), we had moved directly to "what". And we were nowhere near a well thought out implementation method (how).

A public relations crisis made the false start obvious. Although never proven, rumours circulated that some disaffected staff had warned the student union that the stepped care program was a threat to good service. In an effort to save money and decrease wait times, service quality would be compromised. Some clinical staff left the University. They were uncomfortable with the prospect of altering their practices in alignment with the model that was already being adopted. Highly critical articles were published in the student newspaper.

The University communications team became involved. Senior Administration officials had no desire to reverse the course on stepped care—after all, early indications were (contrary to the press reports) that it was working. Secondly, funders were very interested in the model. However, with input from the public relations office, a decision was made to rebrand the change. Instead of stepped care, the new approach was labelled "Cooperative Care". This was a brilliant move because not only would there be a commitment to stepped care principles, but in addition, the issue that had derailed implementation (internal and inter-department conflict) could be addressed with a focus on relationship-building. The crisis became an opportunity to implement a formal process of working through storming at two levels: Level 1 among clinicians and leadership and Level 2 with persons with lived experience (students and the student union leadership).

After the dust settled, it became clear through deliberate engagement with clinicians, student union representatives, as well peer helpers what the problem areas were. The "why change" became more obvious. Students found the current organization of programming confusing. Why were there two departments offering similar services? Which one do I go to? Why do I have to wait so long when we have more funding and more staff than many other colleges and universities? Do we really have quality programming? Can't we do better? By pausing implementation and asking stakeholders whether and/or why anything (whether it be programming, clinical roles or leadership structures) should change, motivation to participate in the design process increased. When the clinicians learned that changes would address inequities in funding between the two units, preserve their professional principles and values through horizontally organized process leadership roles, and that the decisions on how and what to implement would involve them directly, buy-in further increased. Likewise, when the students learned that access to care would be streamlined and the new model would only *add* programming, not remove anything they valued, they were on board. Finally, both groups were reassured that future steps would include consideration of a wide range of possible solutions and that they would be involved in the process. They were invited to search for and create innovations that addressed the issues of importance to them. The fact that staff and students were supported to engage in blue-sky thinking to address their own needs, indicated a shift from why to wow. We had completed Stage 2, identifying *why* change and inspiring some *wow* among the leadership team, clinical staff and the students (persons with lived experience).

7.2.3 Stage 3: Multi-Sectoral Consultations on the Need for Change and Inspiration

We could have stopped at Stage 2. The core stakeholders were engaged. Why do we need to keep moving outward? The University leaders had researched innovations, contracted with us as thought leaders for innovative practice. Students and clinicians were part of the co-design process. Should this not be enough? A wide range of expertise and experience had been tapped. But as Gino cautions, accumulated expertise and experience can be restrictive. In her NPR interview, she referred to a study she conducted on cardiac surgeons who had been notified by the Food and Drug Administration that a routine technique was no longer considered safe. The results indicated that the more experience a surgeon had, the less likely they were to change their practices in response to the FDA warning (Gino, 2018).

The clinicians, managers and students at the University we had worked with thus far had considerable experience. As a result of this experience we wondered if they might be too deep in the forest to recognize out-of-the-box ideas. Compared to outsiders, would their collective years of experience with established practices make them less receptive to novel, experimental ideas? Outsider perspectives, according to Gino, are crucial for innovation.

Following the two suicides at Memorial University (Chap. 3), it was conversations with residence leaders, not counsellors, managers or students attending counselling, that led us to recalibrate what needed to be changed. Before these conversations, the suicide prevention strategy had created an atmosphere of high tension and fear. The risk paradigm had not been challenged. We had not even recognized its presence. The protesting residence leaders alerted me to its presence. And the conversations that followed inspired a vision of a more engaging, vibrant residence community that could be cultivated in the very space occupied by postvention puppies. The idea of bringing fun and games back to that multipurpose room was a *wow* moment. The residence leaders who helped us to see where we were going wrong with the risk paradigm would not have been invited at a Stage 2 level had the distributive design cycle method been in place at Memorial University. But they might be considered for participation as external stakeholders at Stage 3.

At Memorial University, group counselling programming had been poorly attended for years. The student peer network at Memorial could not attract interest in their activities. They had helped to market the groups with us, but with no success. The experts and students with the most experience were stumped. Given the increasing demand and the full waiting rooms, why was there no uptake? We had no answers. But when a new Director of the Botanical Gardens approached me expressing interest in mental health, we discovered an alternative. He had a background working in psychiatric hospitals as a horticultural therapist. He wondered if there might be opportunities for collaborating with the Counselling Centre. He came to a staff meeting and presented on his work. One of our counsellors had expertise in mindfulness. The concept of Green Mindfulness was hatched at this meeting. Together they launched a 90-min weekly walk-in event in a high traffic area of campus. It quickly became known as a place to get a new houseplant. When students wandered in they were invited by students from the peer network to take a cutting and plant it mindfully in a small pot. They were encouraged to feel the texture of soil, its temperature. They could take a mint leaf and absorb the aroma of fresh mint tea. An average of 100 students attended each week. It took an outsider, the Director of the Botanical Gardens, to solve the problem of failed group work and the lack of uptake from peer mentors. Before his appearance, we kept offering the same kind of groups somehow continuing to think people might start coming. The peer mentors, determined to build a successful peer counselling program, continued to host drop-in hours for 2 years despite few takers. None of us considered that we should stop doing this or try something different.

While undoubtedly success stories (bringing fun back to residence and green mindfulness), the prompt for change was random and could easily have been missed. What would have happened if the resident assistant, the director of the Botanical Gardens and all kinds of other outsiders had been deliberately invited to answer the question "why change?" Maybe innovation would have happened more smoothly and rapidly.

Returning to our mid-sized public university, what might the broader community think about change? Would extending the "why change your practices" question be of interest to academic advisors, to the fitness centre, to the student residences, to faculty partners? And then what about the city beyond the campus? Are there no other influential organizations asking questions about change? Could we engage in a broader conversation about change in policies with potential external partners? Who else wants change? Are others being inspired by new ideas? Can we share our "wow" blue sky ideas?

Not surprisingly, conflict also emerged when we got to Stage 3—external stakeholders. Campus staff and faculty invited to participate in the discussion were divided. Some said the problem was that the clinicians were not seeing students fast enough and did not have time to consult with them when they called. Others simply wanted the clinicians to take the mental health problems off their hands; they did not want to learn more about how to support students because that was not part of their job. It appeared that at least one common problem among all stakeholders (clinicians, managers, students, staff and faculty) was the sense of being overloaded with no room to do anything new or more. What were their needs? All stakeholders needed something to make their experiences easier, more manageable and more comfortable. How could *wow* be facilitated for external partners? We already learned that moving too quickly to *how* or *what* will fall flat. Resolving tensions cannot happen without some consensus on the question "why change".

Some tensions were traced to conflicting opinions about what constitutes best practices in mental health care. About a year after implementing Cooperative Care, the Manager of Counselling Services received a complaint from a Student Union Board Member. The Board Member said that students were complaining about the new model. The Manager called the Board Member to suggest they host a joint meeting with all who might have concerns. Several board members attended along with a representative from a student society group focused on mental health awareness programming. The student society representative complained about the quality of care they received at the counselling centre. "What did they say about the quality? Did they have negative experiences?" asked the Counselling Manager. "No", replied the student, "But they both see Dr. X at the health clinic operated by the Faculty of Medicine, and he said to them that they should be getting weekly CBT treatment, with hour-long sessions for up to three months. That is best practice and their symptoms warrant this". The Manager thought for a few moments and then said, "Sometimes care providers on our own teams disagree about what constitutes quality care. If you are interested, I can show you part of a presentation I give frequently which shows how we are both right. CBT is evidence-based but so is our model. Would you like to see what I have been presenting to my colleagues at conferences about our Cooperative Care model?" The students agreed. They asked pointed questions and seemed to leave the meeting both satisfied and intrigued. The Counselling Servicer Manager made a note to set up a meeting with the Chair of Family Medicine.

As external consultations at Stage 3 continued, it turned out there were several philanthropic organizations interested in participating. When they joined, we learned of their concerns about current practices, and more importantly, how eager they were to fund change. For years, these organizations had been funding regional and national projects gathering data in support of innovation. They hinted that some of their funders were now ready to donate large sums of money to support change. Their *raison d'etre* was to fund broad systemic innovations aimed at serving all stakeholders.

They were committed to well thought out strategies based on implementation science. A one-day forum was hosted by one of the philanthropic groups with a focus on implementation science. An expert facilitated the workshop. Participants learned about the drivers of successful design and implementation. They were introduced to tools that would help focus the work at Stages 4, 5 and 6 of the multi-sectoral design cycle. They agreed to engage the implementation science expert again at later stages to support their work.

Prior to the engaging stakeholders on the *why* and *wow* process at Stages 2 and 3, consultations had been reactive and unfocused. Previously, when students or other campus stakeholders complained, or worse, published scathing reports in social media or the campus newspaper, administrators and public relations staff were only able to work on putting out the fires. By the end of Stage 3, however, all parties (the SC2.0 leads, clinicians, managers, persons with lived experience, and external stakeholders) agreed on the *why* of change and were more inspired (*wow*ed) by what could be.

7.2.4 Stage 4: Identify the External Partnerships Their Resources and How to Operationalize Them

With agreement that change was needed and shared understanding of issues to be addressed, all stakeholders were ready to begin identifying solutions. They had been inspired enough by opportunities but there was no agreed upon process for building solutions or a clear sense of what those solutions might look like. It was time for an environmental scan. Field trips were organized. Representatives of the mental health strategy committee arranged visits to three campus that were a little further along in their transformation process. In their visits they asked about their process, the changes, what did and did not work and why. Following the visits, a workshop was held to debrief. Stakeholders at all levels were asked to think about how to move forward. One of the lessons learned by an institution they had visited was to resist the allure of the "shiny object". The Manager of Counselling at one campus they had visited admitted to having a reputation for saying yes to every new and exciting e-mental health program that promised to solve the challenge of increased service demands. While programs were evidence-based or evidence-informed, little attention had been paid to implementation strategy. The utilization rates had been low.

The committee agreed that they did not want to fall into the shiny object trap. One of the members had recently attended a conference where a psychiatrist, now a Canadian Senator, warned that "the bloom will eventually fade and fall off the rose" of e-mental health. While this committee member was not so pessimistic, she was wary of the promise of technology. The hype can be overblown.

The committee struggled with a common implementation tension. One side cried for bold action now, "Mental health reform here is long overdue: we've been working on this forever! One more study will sit on the shelf gathering dust and nothing will change!" While perhaps less passionate, but equally pointed, another committee member countered "Shiny-object syndrome will lead us down blind alleys, we should proceed carefully and cautiously". In the end, they agreed that balance was needed. There might be some things that can be actioned immediately—initiatives that have already been researched and subjected to broad consultation.

Politicians, for better or worse, are masters at balancing quick wins with carefully planned, drawn-out strategies requiring exhaustive consultation. A few carefully selected immediate actions can satisfy pent up demand and inspire others to commit to change. Was there anything in line with their Cooperative Care model that could be implemented without further delay? What needed more careful consideration? A representative from the University's Marketing and Communications department spoke up, "I think what we need is a good communications strategy so that we can leverage anticipation the way Apple does, but of course within an academic values frame". A counsellor on the committee added that managing expectations is very important in mental health treatment; expectations are key to positive outcomes. But she admitted that this was not part of her skillset, and cautioned that, "Our licensing board actually prohibits any type of promotion of psychological services". Due to the potential for manipulating vulnerable persons, advertising is considered unethical.

Another counsellor countered this caution, "We are masters of persuasion. Our practices sell hope. Some psychotherapy schools are explicit in this respect". Ericksonian Hypnotherapy, for example, has influenced many contemporary methods, including solution-focused, narrative, and positive psychology approaches. Has the ethical code proscription on promotion been interpreted too broadly? Other committee members were intrigued. "This could work on so many levels", one said. "The transparency about our process is in keeping with recovery principles. And a more proactive approach could stimulate feelings of anticipation and hope". Perhaps promotion aimed at the principles underlying the system of care would be considered outside the scope of the profession, especially, if it is guided by external partners and administrators and not the practitioners alone. A ripple of excitement spread through the room. The first clear action-step (an example of *what*) was emerging—communications. The committee would work out a full implementation strategy with input from the communications experts sitting on the panel. A communication strategy would roll in tandem with implementation steps.

The committee prepared a report with recommendations organized along six guiding principles: (1) access to care needed to be streamlined—there should be a clear point of entry; (2) options for care need to be expanded since one size does not fit all; (3) the care system needs to be nimble and informed by continuous co-design by all stakeholders; (4) The care system needs to be accountable with its mission to improve outcomes; (5) implementation should follow best practices informed by implementation science; (6) a communications strategy is needed to stimulate hopeful help-seeking.

7.2.5 *Stage 5: Identify Unmet Needs of Students and Adjust Existing Programming and Consider New Ones*

At Stage 5, the work was transferred back to *internal* stakeholders—clinic managers, clinical staff, representatives from Student Affairs and students with lived experience. One of the first tasks was to re-engage with the implementation science consultant. This was deemed essential to ensure the "what" would not get ahead of the "how". Implementation science has been defined as "the scientific study of methods to promote the systematic uptake of research findings and other evidence-based practices into routine practice, and, hence, to improve the quality and effectiveness of health services" (Eccles & Mittman, 2006). The practice has evolved to address what is referred to as "the implementation gap" that exists between research and practice. While evidence may exist to support care practices, the practices are often not adopted. If they are adopted, they may not be used with fidelity to the intervention originally tested. And even if they are used with fidelity to the originally tested intervention, the practices may not be sustained. And if they are sustained in one setting, they may not be scaled up or replicated in other settings. Multiple gaps may interfere with impactful knowledge mobilization.

Our six-stage SC2.0 distributive design cycle is an example of an "active implementation framework" (Metz & Bartley, 2012). In addition to organizing the process through phases that extend across 2–4 years, an active implementation framework specifies useable interventions, drivers for successful implementation, processes for improvement and composition of teams.

An initial step in developing an implementation framework is to articulate a clear description of the program. Second, the essential and gold standard features of a program or model are identified. Third, core interventions are clearly operationalized in line with underlying principles. Finally, practice guidelines and standards are developed to allow for performance and fidelity assessment. Typically, few programs are implemented with attention to all these features of implementation science. While most programs are clearly described, few identify the core or essential components and most fail to operationalize or test for fidelity in practice settings. Our team recently compiled standards for Stepped Care 2.0 in collaboration with the Mental Health Commission of Canada (MHCC, in press). The standards are currently being applied through the implementation of a digital platform that extends SC2.0 to all Canadians as part of the Government of Canada's COVID-19 mental health response (Wellness Together Canada, 2020). The platform provides the technological infrastructure for not only tracking and enhancing outcomes, but also treatment fidelity to the new SC2.0 standards.

As indicated in Fig. 7.1, meaningful outcomes for any new program depend on the efficacy of the intervention, how it is implemented and the context in which implementation occurs. In our six-stage implementation model, enabling contexts are nurtured first by asking *why* change is needed and by inspiring blue-sky *wow* thinking. This nurturing happens long before effective interventions are selected (the *what*) and before application of implementation science (the *how*).

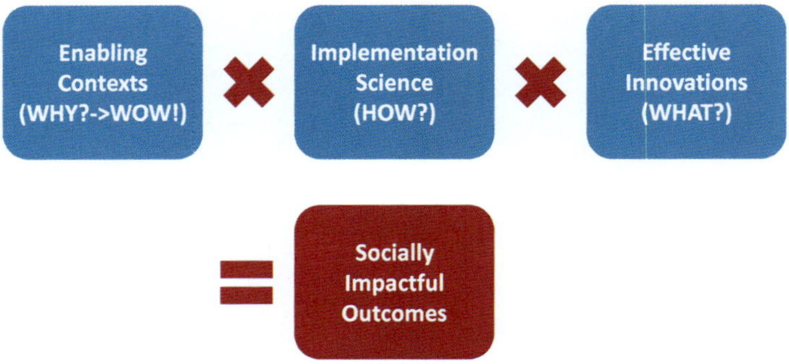

Fig. 7.1 Implementation science outcomes, adapted from National Implementation Research Network (2019)

The Implementation Science consultant met several times with the team. The goal was to develop "useable cooperative" interventions. The University wanted a clear description of what Cooperative Care *really* is. But first the team worked through another full-day workshop aimed at developing Cooperative Care Practice Profiles. Practice profiles were developed using a toolkit designed to operationalize care principles. The toolkit ensured that treatment protocols were based on research and information about best practices. It also ensured that competencies aligned with innovations, and that the innovations would be phased in gradually. It was important that the incremental process of adoption met the expectations of all stakeholders. The facilitator began the day by asking, "What are the critical, non-negotiable components of your cooperative care model? To know if a component is critical, ask yourself, if it were to be missing, would you no longer be able to think of it as Cooperative Care". The team defined cooperative care and came up with five critical components (see Table 7.1).

Then, for each of the five components, workshop participants operationalized, in turn, what ideal implementation, acceptable variations and unacceptable variations might look like. Beside each, they also specified what outcomes could be expected if acceptable variations were applied with fidelity. For example, the first component (flexible approaches) was operationalized first by deciding the number of step categories and then populating them with existing programs. The team decided on a 10-step model ranging from prevention at the lower end to psychiatric consultation at the higher end. But because of the sensitivity to hierarchy, and the long-standing discomfort with the word "stepped care", the category list on their graphic was unnumbered. In the prevention category, four programs were specified: orientation events, outreach/distress activities, training for professors and other campus staff, and departmental talks for the various faculties.

Table 7.1 The core components of "Cooperative Care"

Cooperative Care means that our healthcare professionals work with students and explore various services to find the best kind of care for their needs. This means using one or multiple treatment options, both traditional and holistic. Our staff collaborates with campus colleagues, other care providers, peers and community services to support students and meet their individual needs. Cooperative Care includes:
1. **Flexible** approaches that match students with the right resource at the right time to help students feel better—fast.
2. **Treatment that gives students choices**, building on their existing strengths and autonomy.
3. **Community-based care** that pulls together resources on-campus, off-campus and online, depending on what best fits students' needs.
4. **A holistic wellness approach** that targets all of the factors that contribute to overall student wellness.
5. **Goal-oriented care** that builds resiliency and focuses on what makes them well rather than only discussing what makes them unwell.

The second component (treatment that gives students choices) was operationalized in several ways. One stemmed from a mock webpage storyboard created by participants to map out the envisioned help-seeker experience. They drafted a Counselling Services webpage with the title: "What kind of support are you looking for?" Four top-level options were drafted (1) mental health support; (2) support for a physical health condition; (3) academic support; (4) I want to learn more about mental health and self-care. If the student were to click on the first option (mental health support), three options would appear: (a) I need to speak with someone right now; (b) It's not a crisis but I still need to talk; (c) I am not in immediate distress or I am open to online resources. Then if the student were to choose option 2 (it's not a crisis but I still need to talk), they would see four options: speaking to a professional right now, speaking to a professional in person, speak to a peer, or speak to an academic advisor.

By the end of the day, practice profiles were completed for all five components of the Cooperative Care Model. Participants were cautioned that none of these operationalized care components would succeed without careful attention to enabling factors. What needed to be in place to support implementation? What were the implementation drivers for their campus? These were identified at the next meeting. As indicated in Fig. 7.2, several drivers were specified on organizational, leadership and competency dimensions. On the organizational level, support was needed to adapt policy, fund new initiatives, support the implementation process, and develop technological infrastructure. Managers had to develop new procedures for operations, and strategies for anticipating and mitigating team dysfunction that might arise through the transformation process. Clinical and organizational training was needed to adapt practices and develop new competencies. A system of coaching or mentoring was needed to support ongoing adjustments to care.

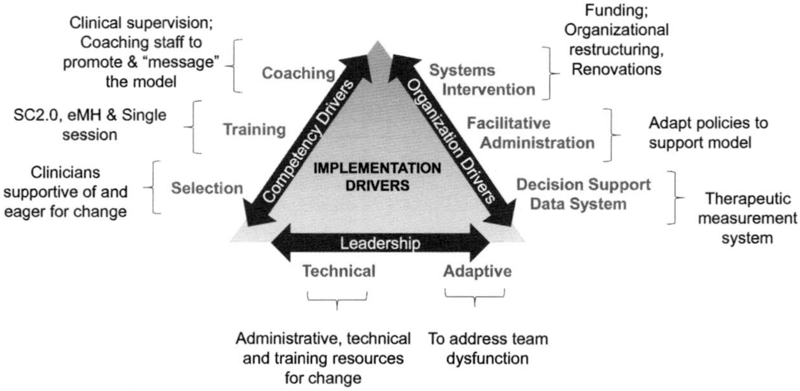

Fig. 7.2 Implementation drivers, adapted from National Implementation Research Network (2019)

7.2.6 *Stage 6: Re-allocate Resources to Support Adjustments and Procure New Programs*

At Stage 6, the co-design process was complete. The Implementation Team was in full operation, useable interventions had been defined and enabling structures were in place. Funding from donors had been received and matched by the University. Architects and contractors were hired to redesign and renovate the space to facilitate smooth, integrated, cooperative care. Technological infrastructure for self-check-ins, shared record-keeping, therapeutic monitoring and web-page improvements was developed. Policies and procedures were adapted or created anew.

New staff with experience in walk-in, single-session counselling, and e-mental health care were recruited and hired. None of these new staff were hired within the existing counsellor collective bargaining unit. This decision was made in collaboration with the union representing counsellors. Vacancies within the bargaining unit would continue to be filled for the next 3 years and hiring outside of the bargaining unit could only be made with new funds. This agreement helped resolve some of the anxiety expressed by existing staff about the future of their roles. On the other hand, it meant that some of the existing staff no longer felt obligated to adjust their practices in line with the new Cooperative Care model, since this new way of practicing was only required by the new hires outside of the bargaining unit. We reminded the managers of the units to use the same approach to change management as counsellors use with their clients in the context SC2.0. Rather than urging staff to become more ready for change, the job of managers was to connect with staff where they were already.

This pivot to where people are ready did not mean that any staff would be isolated from the new model. Training was provided to all staff on recovery principles, stepped care decision-making, collaborative care, walk-in care interviewing techniques, case management and e-mental health tool use. Weekly meeting agenda structures were adapted to facilitate modified operations. For example, case conferences shifted focus to sharing successes and failures with single session care, stepping decisions, therapeutic monitoring and using time more flexibly. Staff were supported to join community of practice webinars on stepped care, attend relevant conferences and conduct research on topics related to the new model.

At the time of writing, Stage 6 implementation had just begun. The renovations were complete, and a more centralized, collaborative care hub was in operation. A flatter organizational structure was in place with six leads reporting to a new Assistant Dean of Campus Wellness. The two mental health managers, as well as the manager of primary care services, had received promotions to campus lead roles. There was still a lot of work to do before the new Wellness Hub would be truly integrated. The physicians were still operating in isolation and there was no unified health record. A new cycle of design would be needed to move to fully collaborative care.

7.3 Adaptations at Other Sites

There are infinite ways to develop stepped care. Some of the earliest adopters of SC2.0 organize their programming in a non-hierarchical pattern. The University of British Columbia was one of the first Canadian institutions to adapt the model from our campus. As indicated in Fig. 7.3, programming is still arranged in linear fashion but there is no implied hierarchy. Arranged horizontally, there is no suggestion that one program is better than the other. In consultations following introduction to

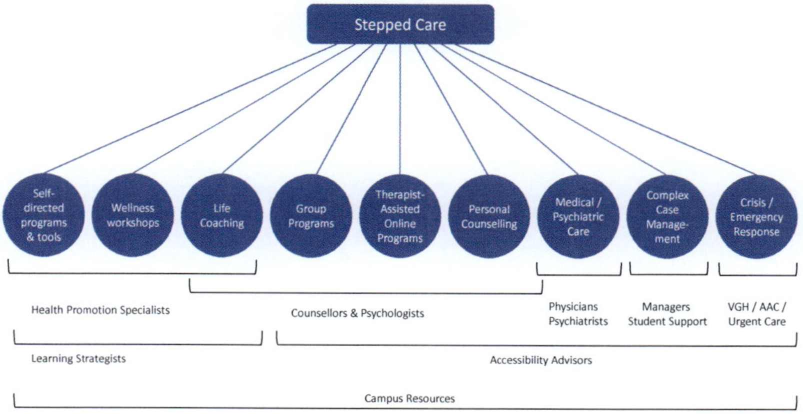

Fig. 7.3 University of British Columbia's adaptation of SC2.0 (Cornish, 2019)

SC2.0, some stakeholders expressed discomfort with the values associated with the three dimensions (i.e. on the x, y, and z axes). One worry was that help-seekers might feel cheated with lower intensity programs or with programs requiring less investment. The arrangement along the continuums might reinforce the prevailing assumption that psychiatric care or face-to-face intensive psychotherapy is more valuable or more effective. If this were the case, help-seekers might be less inclined to consider low-intensity program offerings.

Other non-linear versions of SC2.0 are more explicit. Instead of arranging steps perpendicularly along the x or y axes, interventions are positioned around a circle. The Province of Newfoundland and Labrador now organizes publicly funded mental healthcare for adults into seven categories which are arranged in a circle around the help-seeker. This emphasizes their commitment to client-centric care, in which the help-seeker preferences are accommodated as much as possible. Following consultation with us, The George Washington University in Washington DC and Algonquin College in Ottawa have also developed circular versions of SC2.0. The Newfoundland and Labrador version is still under development. The two other circular versions are illustrated in Fig. 7.4.

The importance of client-centricity cannot be overstated. Helen (a pseudonym), is a local hero in my mind. She is the the CEO of Newfoundland and Labrador's only Province-wide peer network (CHANNAL), literally lives recovery principles. Helen is a person with lived experience who continues to struggle from time to time, but somehow manages to break new ground on multiple fronts. Amber's story in Chap. 4 is a testament to Helen's impact. Helen coined one of my favourite recovery phrases: "ATP, ask the person first!" she exclaims with the broadest of smiles. This refrain is a constant reminder to all of us working on mental health reform. Before making any prescriptions based expert opinion why not simply "ask the person"

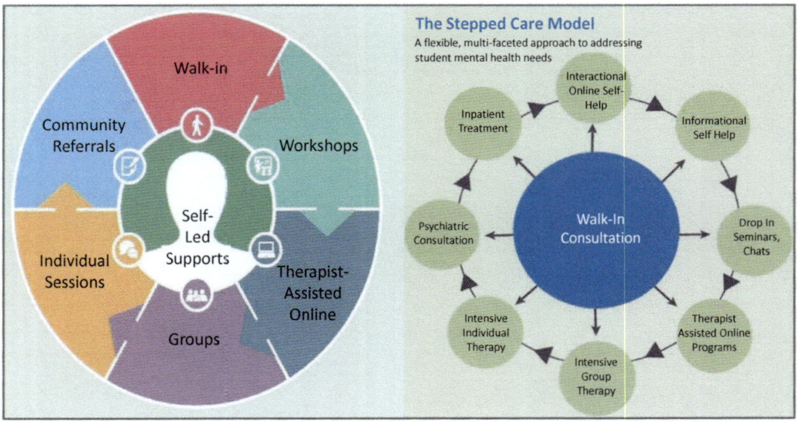

Fig. 7.4 Variations on SC2.0 (from left to right): Algonquin College, the George Washington University (Cornish, 2019)

first? Helen says this with such good humour, and so often, that the acronym, ATP is now common parlance in the Province's mental health sector.

Circles are ancient features of healing practices. Sacred circles have a long tradition throughout the world. When people gather in a circle, they are practicing connection, equality, sustainability and unity. If there is power expressed, it is not a power-*over* anyone or anything. Instead it is power-*with*. The Medicine Wheel, a term coined by people of European descent, is a common structure for organizing knowledge in North American Indigenous populations. The Earth's resources and habitats, if preserved in their natural state, have healing power. The resource configuration across the four quadrants (North, East, South and West) of the wheel represents the natural order of our planet, Mother Earth (Fig. 7.5). Order is not forced. It is what was there to begin with. Wellness and harmony are achieved by aligning with the balancing forces of nature, the elements, the four directions and the cycle of life. While sacred circles bear some resemblance to our SC2.0 circular stepped care models, we are careful to avoid cultural appropriation. We aspire to anti-oppressive and anti-colonial values and avoid making firm assumptions of relevance to Indigenous peoples and their communities. If invited, however, we would welcome opportunities for co-design.

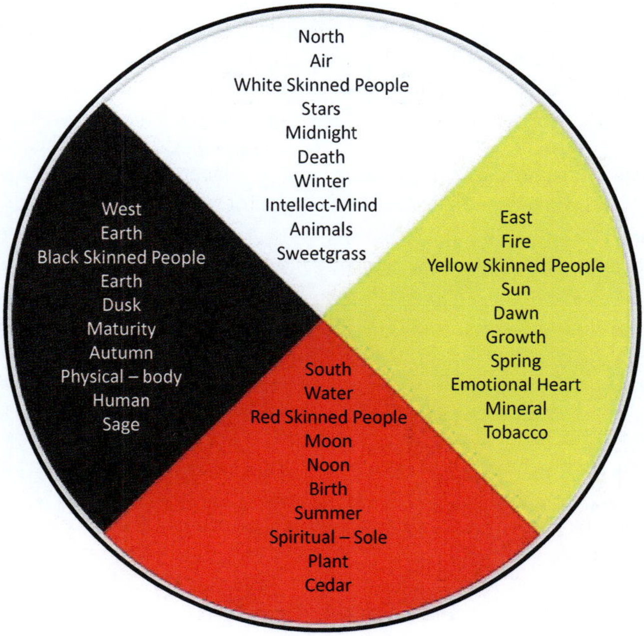

Fig. 7.5 The medicine wheel (Indigenous Corportate Training Inc., 2019)

Foxes and Hedgehogs

Francesca Gino might consider me an aspiring rebel leader. I still have a lot to learn though. My humble attempts to lead have yielded mixed results. I broke the rules and while I did attract a following, I left my team behind. Good rebel leaders practice humility. They make themselves vulnerable through risk-taking. And with the right balance of positive deviance, good judgement, tact and empathy, they manage to bring others with them. There is a tension between disruption, collaboration and nurturing. Effective rebel leadership requires the right mix of bold action and patience. Perhaps a more reasonable approach is to assemble a flat rebel leadership team with complementary collegial roles. I am good at positive deviance but not so good at nurturing. Our Stepped Care Solutions social enterprise has some of these qualities. We have systems thinkers and concrete thinkers. We have peacemakers and disruptors. We have salespeople and we have deviants. I am reminded of a conversation many years ago with my doctoral thesis supervisor who spoke of foxes and hedgehogs. He identified with the fox and wondered if I did too. According to the Ancient Greek poet, Archilochus, "The fox knows many things, but the hedgehog knows one big thing". Hedgehogs burrow down, espousing a single, grand idea to explain everything, while foxes run around on the surface coming up with new ideas to fit every separate encounter. Isiah Berlin popularized this distinction, but later regretted the overly simple dichotomous interpretations of his 1953 essay. I still don't know which I am. I think it is a dialectic. I strive for the grand idea—SC2.0, but the idea itself is amorphous. It slips and slides through co-design, a built-in disruptive process.

We need bold thinking. We need humility. We need risk-takers. We need caretakers. The fable of the fox and the cat (Aesop, 1893) *is a variation on the fox/hedgehog dichotomy. The fox and the cat discuss their varied talents, namely their tricks and dodges in the face of danger. The fox has many, whereas the cat admits to just one plan. When hunters arrive, the cat immediately flees to the safety of high tree branches. The fox can't decide, thinks of many options, and tries a few but none with commitment. The fox is caught by the hounds. In this perilous context, the fox fails and pays with its life. Mass media reports warn that we are in the midst of a mental health crisis. Risk managers, in efforts to maintain reputations of insurers, insist on a cat-like, focused and rigid protocol. Professional associations for the most part follow suit. Does the cat plan save lives? While the cat survives, we can't all hide in trees. A risk averse approach to mental healthcare protects providers more than those they serve. Help seekers are frustrated by this overly cautious approach. Do they want only foxes? Probably not. Isiah Berlin wouldn't either. Why not dispel with dichotomies. We need cats, hedgehogs, and foxes. Cats climb up to watch out for danger. Hedgehogs focus on details. Foxes run around practicing sly deviance and disruption. Let's make room for all three.*

References

Aesop. (1893). The fox and the cat. In E. Grisit (ed.), *Aesop's fables* (p. 193). London: Cassell & Company. https://play.google.com/books/reader?id=ezkSkOjcoGkC&hl=en&pg=GBS.PR1

Cornish, P. (2019, December 13). *Variants on stepped care 2.0.* Retrieved from Stepped Care 2.0: Collaborating for Mental Health Innovation: https://steppedcaretwopoint0.ca/variants-on-stepped-care-2-0/

Eccles, M. P., & Mittman, B. S. (2006). Welcome to implementation science. *Implementation Science, 1*(1), 1–3.

Indigenous Corportate Training Inc. (2019, December 4). *What is an Aboriginal medicine wheel?* Retrieved from Working Effectively with Indigenous Peoples Blog: https://www.ictinc.ca/blog/what-is-an-aboriginal-medicine-wheel

Gino, F. (2018, July 23). *You 2.0: Rebel with a cause.* (S. Vedantam, Interviewer) NPR. Retrieved November 30, 2019, from https://www.npr.org/2018/07/23/631524581/you-2-0-rebel-with-a-cause

Metz, A., & Bartley, L. (2012). *Active implementation frameworks for program success: How to use implementaiton science to improve outcomes for children.* Frank Porter Graham Child Development Institute, National Implementation Research Network. Chapel Hill: Frank Porter Graham Child Development Institute. Retrieved January 2, 2020, from https://static1.squarespace.com/static/5279554ce4b0eea3e5bdac41/t/5bfd5e1a2b6a28d7b076a437/1543331355258/1a_NIRN_ImpArticle.pdf

MHCC (in press). *Stepped Care 2.0 (Revised) Implementation Guide.* Mental Health Commission of Canada. Ottawa, ON.

National Implementation Research Network. (2019, December 13). *Active implementation formula.* Retrieved from https://nirn.fpg.unc.edu/module-3/topic-3/function-3

Sinek, S. (2009). *Start with why: How great leaders inspire everyone to take action.* London: Penguin.

Wellness Together Canada. (2020, May 20). *Wellness Together Canada: Mental Health and Substance Use Support.* Retrieved from Wellness Together Canada: Mental Health and Substance Use Support: https://ca.portal.gs/

Chapter 8
Towards a Paradigm Shift

Contents

You've Turned My World Upside-Down

When we are invited to consult on mental health service or system transformation, we typically try to meet with a wide variety of stakeholder groups to explore their ideas of what works and what doesn't. Usually, I begin by describing what I have learned in my own work and how this has evolved into the SC2.0 model. I outline what is unique about SC2.0 with an emphasis on recovery principles, moving beyond the deficit model and incorporating more open access to a broader range of supports. At a recent invited visit to a West-coast campus psychiatry clinic, I noticed a wide-eyed stare from a psychiatry resident as she listened to me describe the model. There was a moment of silence before she said bluntly but without any judgement, "Everything you have said today contradicts all that I have been taught during my psychiatry residency". While she seemed shocked, I noted an element of wonder and curiosity in her tone of voice. Something clicked. Emotion was aroused. These are the kinds of moments we need to capture to mobilize a paradigm shift. There is confusion, some conflict with what had been thought of as tried and true, and yet a glimmer of hope that a bold new approach could be refreshing.

8.1 SC2.0 Today

SC2.0 is a flexible system for reforming mental healthcare. It supplies scaffolding for organizing and selecting from among best practices, informal supports and new and emerging illness prevention, health promotion and treatment methods. Two meanings of the word "system" drawn from the Oxford English Dictionary (OED Online n.d.) apply to SC2.0:

P. Cornish, *Stepped Care 2.0: A Paradigm Shift in Mental Health*,
https://doi.org/10.1007/978-3-030-48055-4_8

1. A group or set of related or associated things perceived or thought of as a unity or complex whole.
2. An organized scheme or plan of action, esp. one of a complex or comprehensive kind; an orderly or regular method of procedure, government, administration, etc.

Note that the first definition is not prescriptive. It is simply a group of related things organized into a complex whole. Unlike the second definition, it is silent on application or plan of action. We have not yet decided which definition is best suited to SC2.0. While it is tempting to jump to the second plan-of-action definition, it conflicts with the post-modern plurality of values and techniques associated with recovery strategies. If no one size fits all, what is the value of prescribing? On the other hand, what use is a nicely organized group of ideas or principles without recommendations for action. I propose a dialectic. It is important to oscillate among the parts of the system. In our distributive design cycle method we move back and forth from theory or principles to prescription. In keeping with the values of co-design and evolving cultural plurality, prescriptions are bound to fail. The action plan will be abandoned forcing a return to pure values. The failure might also prompt a reworking of the principles. This iterative process is like the qualitative research method of Grounded Theory (Charmaz, 2014). With this method, theory is continuously discovered using constant comparison of concepts and the data they represent. With every new data point observed, the capacity of the concept to represent is reviewed. Each interpretation and finding are compared with existing findings as they emerge from the data analysis. With a finite data set, the iterative process from data to theory evolves to the point at which insights from the process have been exhausted. There is no final data set for mental health practice. As such the iterative process between application and theory is a constant.

Systems are rooted in principles. A principle has been defined as "a fundamental truth or proposition on which others depend; a general statement or tenet forming the (or a) basis of a system of belief, or a primary assumption forming the basis of a chain of reasoning" (OED Online n.d.). Here are the principles, underlying SC2.0 as we understand them today:

1. To maximize impact, a broad continuum of programming – including self-managed resources, family/community/peer support and professional services – matched to readiness, preference, and need is offered, for example:
   (a) Low intensity.
   (b) Same-day access.
   (c) E-mental health.
   (d) Multiple modalities (in person, phone, web).
   (e) Therapy one-at-a-time.
2. Recovery principles and collaborative, co-created wellness plans are incorporated in all therapeutic encounters.
3. Therapeutic measurement is for users and must be part of every care encounter.

4. An agile, flexible, responsive model, co-designed with persons with lived experience must be represented graphically so that the entire system and its parts can be viewed at a glance.

Representing the model graphically, as described in the fourth principle, ensures transparency. A recovery-based model is only as useful as it is visible. A graphical representation allows stakeholders to see the forest *and* the trees. It is equally important for stakeholders to see the many distinct relevant options as it is to see the big picture or to discern an overall pattern from this mass of detail. Preference is viable only if informed by the principles that organize the elements into a whole. Informed choice requires an understanding of how each option is distinguishable from the others and relates to the system organizing principles.

8.2 Synergy and Culture

Two psychologists have influenced my work in lasting ways. John Conway was my supervisor for both my Master's and Doctoral theses. Richard (Dick) Katz sat on both committees as an advisor. While both John and Dick were more foxes than hedgehogs (see Chap. 7), Dick focused on Indigenous healing; whereas John had no one true calling. John is, perhaps, what Career Coach Emilie Wapnick calls a *multipotentialite*. He has had many interests, jobs and interlocking potentials. John, now retired, was a psychologist and a photographer. He was interested in personality, humanism, and social activism. He was comfortable supervising students like me, whose interests were both broad and idiosyncratic. John was a generalist and as such did not believe he needed to play the expert role when supervising. Instead he gently guided exploration and discovery. Dick started his career at Harvard at the time of Timothy Leary and Richard Alpert. Those were heady days. He spent 2 years compiling an ethnographic study of the Kalahari!Kung tribe in Botswana and has become a leading scholar in Indigenous healing psychology (Katz, 2017). He introduced me to the concept of synergy.

Buckminster Fuller was another multipotentialite. He was an architect, systems theorist, designer and inventor most famous for his work on geodesic domes. I grew up in Montreal. I was 4 years old in 1967 when my birth city hosted the World's Fair. The feature that most impressed me at the time (besides the punching balloons distributed for free at the gate) was the American Pavilion (named the Biosphere), a giant geodesic dome designed by Fuller. According to Fuller, synergy means "the behaviour of whole systems unpredicted by the behaviour of their parts taken separately" (Fuller, 1975). Admittedly less elegant than the structures he is famous for, this definition can be rephrased as the whole is greater than the sum of the parts. A geodesic dome is made of up of thousands of simple tubes of metal, which on their own have limited strength or potential. But arranged in the shape of a dome, they form what engineers claim is the most efficient and robust structure imaginable.

Domes are lightweight but almost indestructible. Fuller's Biosphere is still there despite bursting into flames during minor renovations in 1976. It is now a Museum dedicated to promoting the environment and its protection.

Dick Katz applies the concept of synergy to distinguish ancient Indigenous healing practices from those of modern Eurocentric medicine (Katz, 2017). In the context of Western medicine, healing resources are scarce, expensive and difficult to access. In the context of our capitalist economy, scarce resources are highly valued and their value can only be maintained if the supply is either naturally or intentionally limited. The cost of years of required specialized training ensures that Western medicine will retain its rare commodity status. Ancient Indigenous healing resources, Katz argues, are plentiful and because these resources belong to everyone, their potential is virtually unlimited. Everyone in the community brings healing potential. And when those healing resources are welcomed and arranged with care, they take on the synergistic power of a geodesic dome. This is a power *with* others. It literally takes a village.

My vision for SC2.0 has been inspired by the concept of synergy. There are almost endless parts; unlimited options for supporting mental health. If these are arranged thoughtfully, they can create a powerful and sustainable system of mental health. Each part alone is limited, but when connected, integrated and held in balance, healing is perpetuated. If one small part, one tube fails, the remaining pieces keep the structure intact. Failing forward is possible. If a specialist is not available for months, a peer-support person can make the wait more meaningful. Waiting is no longer unproductive. The structure ensures endless support.

It is easy to get lost in complex systems. By bringing together so many parts SC2.0 can get messy and tangled. I am no stranger to this. I am the first to admit that my nine-step graphical representation of SC2.0 is a little short on elegance. True also for the Distributive Design Cycle introduced in Chap. 6. I need a little more parsimony. Perhaps it is not surprising that we can find some of the most elegant structures featured in the longest surviving human cultural communities. The igloo is a dome made from the (once) most ubiquitous material—ice. Tragically, it is now becoming a scarce commodity. The T-Pee is another elegant structure. A few poles and animal skin. Both natural, sustainable materials that are used frugally and efficiently. The structure is portable allowing for movement across the land. And with that movement the land recovers so that it may continue to sustain life.

Can SC2.0 be inspired by this ancient wisdom? It is still too early to tell. I have, admittedly appropriated this knowledge. My intent is to engage with Indigenous peoples and elders when the time is right. When I am invited to do so. Their voices are needed to further inform the transformation process.

8.3 Frugal Innovation

Navi Radjou has spent years studying "jugaad" or frugal innovation. He defines it simply as "doing more with less". Radjou puts an environmental sustainability spin on his call for "global innovation networks" to "create more business and social value while minimizing the use of diminishing resources such as energy, capital and time". Ironically while globalization has lifted many out of poverty in developing nations including Radjou's native India, it has also accelerated climate change and eroded the middle class in developed nations, widening the gap between rich and poor. Not surprisingly, critics smell a rat. Frugal innovation is the latest chapter in neo-liberal policies that shift the cost burden to consumers and lend support to public and private austerity measures. And somehow the rich still get richer. Radjou's next forthcoming book, *Conscious Society: Reinventing How We Consume, Work and Live*, expected in 2021 will extend frugal innovation to lifestyle (Radjou, 2020).

Innovation often has both bright and dark sides. An improvement is an opportunity that can distribute benefit or withhold it. In the case of SC2.0, some critics argue that the model enables funders to divert investment in mental health by cutting expensive specialist care and shifting labour to less expensive technological or "cost-free" alternatives such as peer and family support. Insurance companies will retain cash that can be invested in stocks and their own bottom lines. I am under no illusions; there is no doubt that this incentive is driving corporate decision-making. However, savvy business leaders have been aware of high return on investment in mental health spending for longer than their public sector and academic counterparts. Investment in mental health will not consume scarce resources or damage the environment. Better partnerships between public and private sectors are needed to ensure that everyone wins. Social and corporate enterprise can co-exist. Vibrant social democracies in Europe have proven that partnerships between labour, industry and government work. There does not have to be a loser. It is time to abandon the zero-sum, divisive, confrontational North American scarcity-based paradigm in favour of a more collaborative, synergistic paradigm.

Mental health care has long been the purview of elites. It was this way in Victorian times and not much has changed. In his 1964 book, *Psychotherapy: The Purchase of Friendship*, psychologist William Schofield suggested the profession is biased towards treating only those who are young, attractive, verbal, intelligent and successful (or YAVIS). What has changed? Cheaper psycho-pharmaceuticals with less adverse side effects have extended the reach of treatment, but psychotherapy is still only accessible to those with privilege. If anything, what has changed is that we have a greater appreciation of how psychotherapy privileges the *white, heterosexual* YAVIS population. While we are not there yet, one of my goals with SC2.0 is that we might finally release the power and potential of mental health innovation to benefit the whole population.

8.4 Evolution or Revolution

My colleague and friend, Gillian Berry, has written a chapter to be published in the next SC2.0 book in the series. She said she wants to call it "Why SC2.0 Won't Work". That's okay, I thought. She's a disruptor too. Gillian is of Caribbean descent. Her ancestors were slaves transplanted to what is now British Ghiana. She was born and raised in England and now lives in the United States. She was the first to implement SC2.0 in the United States at the George Washington University Counseling Center. Her approach was bold. On 31 August 2015, the triple digit wait-list was eliminated. Overnight she and her team introduced a same-day, walk-in only access system. Students at this large, private, expensive university were pleased with the model. While some staff struggled at first and there was a fair amount of turnover, the staff who remained and those who were subsequently hired could not imagine turning back.

Back to Gillian's title. As a woman of colour and descendent of slaves, Gillian is sceptical of any promise of reform. "The entire system is broken and rigged against us!" she exclaims. "How can you even imagine this will make a difference?" True, I think. Paradigm shifts are rare. Evolution is slow. Revolutions seldom succeed. Gillian is undoubtedly a rebel leader, but she cannot afford to be as idealistic as me. Idealism is easy for a white, middle-aged, educated male.

I was surprised and delighted to learn soon after I first met Gillian, that she, like Dick Katz had spent time in Botswana where she, too, learned about Indigenous healing from the Kalahari!Kung peoples. Gillian incorporates this ancient wisdom, practiced by her ancestors into her practice with many of her marginalized clients. The practices are not privileged. They are accessible and empowering. It is a power-*with* others. They speak truth to hegemonic power. But in the end, on their own or in the context of SC2.0, it won't spark a revolution.

8.5 SC2.0 Tomorrow

This book is the first in a series of three. It is different in tone and sentiment. It is somewhat autobiographical. I share the thoughts, musings and experiences of my journey into mental healthcare disruption. Books 2 and 3 are more academic in content and structure. Both are edited volumes with a wide range of contributors. Book 2 questions almost everything I have written in this book. In true disruptor fashion, it aims to tear it all down in order to build it up better. And that is where Book 3 picks it up. After some rigorous critique, what are we left with? What do we know? Where can we go?

Book 2 begins with a recap of book 1. Chapter 2 is an academic scoping review of the existing literature on stepped care. The working title, *Stepped Care Research Findings: A Dog's Breakfast or Enough to Move Forward,* summarizes the broader research literature on stepped care (not just SC2.0). As dedicated health researchers, the authors of the chapter reflect on the challenges and frustrations associated with translating or mobilizing research findings to produce meaningful policy or mental health system reform. The third chapter, written by a counsellor (who is also a lawyer), questions the risk paradigm and how it dominates both our society and our mental healthcare system, restricting practices with the intention to reduce liability and defend institutional reputation. For readers who are practitioners, the chapter touches the sense of loss they feel when regulations and risk-averse policymakers stifle creative therapeutic innovations. It encourages them to gently rise-up in the interest of healthcare reform and the development of a more meaningful work setting. The fourth chapter explores a key distinction of the SC2.0 model, one that raises questions about the nature of evidence, especially evidence relevant to quality mental healthcare. Specifically, the authors debate each other in this chapter on the relative merits of specific and non-specific treatment factors, including whether practice-based evidence (i.e. monitoring the impact after the fact on a case-by-case basis) is more likely to maximize positive outcomes than rigorous implementation of evidence-based treatments. The final chapter in book 2, Section I is Gillian's (described above). It raises questions about the fit or relevance of current models of care for marginalized groups. It delves into varied cultural values and sociological theory, exploring the potential of SC2.0 for addressing marginalization and post-colonial trauma while cautioning on limits set by socio-economic inequities. Berry provocatively concludes, SC2.0 won't work for marginalized peoples, but admits with some hesitation that it is the best we can come up with at least without a full-fledged revolution!

Book 2, Section II introduces initial implementation experiences of early adopters. Chapter 6 begins with the authors' disparate stories of frustration and despair experienced with a flawed care system prior to implementation. Then some connections, curiosity and glimpses of hope emerge alongside clues for shifting their work. A eureka moment explodes, and they launch forth with a bold transformation of the care system literally overnight. Chapter 7 insists that narrative therapy and solution-focused single-session (or therapy one-at-a-time) principles are foundational to SC2.0 while at the same time produce a vexing tension. On the one hand, this approach can bring the kind of dramatic rapid access changes described in the previous chapter. But on the other hand, the stepped care continuum itself dilutes the magic of single session by hinting people really might need more. The authors engage in some friendly intellectual discourse on this dialectic. Several well-published authors on single-session practices, increasingly adopted across Canada and the United States, make cameo text-box appearances to enliven the debate. Chapter 8 tests the metal of the model. Can it meet the needs of those with disabilities? How flexible is it? Should one declare a disability, seek accommodations, or muscle through? What do recovery principles say to this? The author ponders these questions reflecting on his personal experience with dyslexia as well as his work supporting students with disabilities. Chapter 9 describes adaptations of SC2.0 at a variety of post-secondary institutions and community mental health settings across North America. Through a discussant format, this chapter captures or recreates the essence and content of some lively debates on SC2.0 hosted at live panels over the past 2 years. It questions whether the transformations inspired by SC2.0 are variations of a single distinct model or examples of organic, independent systems relevant only to local contexts. Chapter 10 closes by setting the stage for the third, yet more detailed book on implementation. The chapter previews some of the enablers and obstacles to adoption of the model and describes some promising areas of research and application under development.

The third book in the series digs deep into implementation science, beginning with a recap of the first two books. The second chapter provides an overview of implementation science theory. Co-design, communication and marketing are key drivers for successful implementation. Chapter 3 describes the recovery model of mental healthcare and summarizes research. SC2.0 implementation case material is provided to illustrate application. Key recovery principles include consumer involvement in design and strengths-based programming focused on functioning. Chapter 4 reviews resilience and flourishing research and describes how these constructs are being operationalized in SC2.0 therapeutic measurement (e.g. assessing functioning and flourishing) and interventions based on positive psychology. Chapter 5 describes how the concepts of scarcity and synergy can explain the structure of formal versus informal healthcare systems. A scarcity paradigm has dominated Western-based medical approaches, whereas synergy is a hallmark of ancient more traditional healing practices. The scarcity paradigm holds that valuable health resources are scarce and must be rationed. The synergy paradigm suggests that healing resources, more broadly defined, are unlimited and that by integrating the many varied simple components of healing, the whole is greater than the sum of the parts. Healing resources expand with integration. By considering together the implementation of both population-health and clinic-based programming, it becomes possible without the silos for policy makers to determine through a holistic lens an optimal mix of illness prevention, wellness promotion and clinical interventions. Finally, some providers and policy-makers question whether SC2.0 implementation aligns with professional codes and treatment guidelines. Chapter 6 reasons that SC2.0 practice can improve adherence to ethical guidelines for licensed counsellors, social workers and psychologists.

With principles and strategies for implementation outlined in Section I, the reader is ready for broader application of the model described in Sect. II. Chapter 7 defines low-intensity programming and dispels myths that dissuade some practitioners and clients from adopting the principle of trying simple first. One myth is that low-intensity programming, including e-mental health, is only appropriate for people with mild or moderate concerns. This is discriminatory. A person with severe symptoms can benefit as much or more from peer support, even some e-mental health tools. Readiness and functioning are generally independent of illness severity. Chapter 8 challenges professionals to widen the tent of clinical care to include. Or, at least legitimize both formal and informal community-based supports. This can be done through social prescriptions, followed by careful comparative monitoring of these programs alongside more formal traditional interventions. Chapter 9 examines the dialectical decision-making process associated with group versus individual programming referrals. A group might be the treatment of choice for social anxiety, but clients may not be prepared for the high dosage of anxiety associated with social exposure. In this case, group is a higher intensity program—a high dose with correspondingly high side effects for the client, but a less resource-intensive option for the provider. Alternatively, a workshop. At Step 4 is both less intensive and less expensive. Chapter 10 invites policy and decision-makers to consider the SC2.0 framework for organizing both clinic and population-based interventions as one system. This only makes sense given that the end user is both a patient and not a patient and may rightly see no distinction. Chapter 11 illustrates how SC2.0 can serve as scaffolding for organizing complimentary roles of professionals from (a) varied clinical disciplines and (b) other sectors that include educators, first responders, clergy, Indigenous healers and peer-support workers. Chapter 13 is a call for partnerships with industry to draw on the potential for big data analytics to inform care decisions and choices among all the SC2.0 options. The promise of continuous quality improvement is alluring. Chapter 14 closes the volume with questions about even broader application through the entire healthcare space. There really is no health system currently. Could there be?

Neo-Liberal Ruse

AnnMarie Churchill is a colleague who has been working closely with me on implementation and evaluation of SC2.0. She has a Master's degree in Social Work and a Doctorate in Experimental Psychology. Like me, she is a rebel leader and a systems thinker. It seemed like a slam dunk when she applied for a tenure-track position at Memorial University's School of Social Work. She has decades of experience of training and social justice work with Indigenous populations, she is a fierce critic of systems and hierarchies. While she made it to the last round of interviews, the search committee did not recommend her for the position. The rumour was that her involvement with SC2.0 disqualified her. The faculty were suspicious. The model is just a neo-liberal ruse for reducing public investment in mental health by outsourcing to private industry (e-mental health vendors) and offloading care to peer supporters and informal (free) community-based networks. The assumption was that SC2.0 was a way to do less with less.

I was not as surprised to see similar critiques from my colleagues on the listserv of the Association of University College and Counseling Center Directors. Most of the directors are counsellors or clinical psychologists by training. Disruption and social justice are not central to the curriculum. Some of the responses were predictable: "Stepped Care is a threat to our profession. It will erode the quality of our counselling and psychotherapy thereby short-changing students with inferior low-intensity care. It is the beginning of the end of our professions especially when we start to outsource to fly-by-night e-mental health vendors driven only by profits." I was also not surprised to see critiques from colleagues in my own backyard. I received a copy of an email from a psychologist in Atlantic Canada who accused me of being a "shameless self-promoter". Shameless disrupter, yes, but self-promoter?

The fears expressed by colleagues in all mental health disciplines are well-founded. We know all too well that fear transforms into defensive anger when solutions cannot be found. The dangers are real. Neo-liberal forces are at work.

Neo-conservative populism is another threat. Both work to erode investment in the public good for the benefit of elites. I don't want to be duped by these forces. Good rebel leaders watch their backs and maintain healthy scepticism. My three grown children help me in this respect. My youngest is training to be an environmental chemist. She will save the planet. My middle child is an environmental geologist. She will fight the fossil fuel industry. My son, the eldest is a legal aid lawyer fighting for the homeless and illegal migrants. My son said to me about this book and SC2.0: "It's not going to do anything for my clients". Gillian might agree. It's still too YAVIS.

References

Charmaz, K. (2014). *Constructing grounded theory* (2nd ed.). Los Angeles: Sage.

Fuller, B. (1975). *Synergetics: Explorations in the geometry of thinking*. New York: MacMillan.

Katz, R. (2017). *Indigenous healing psychology: Honoring the wisdom of the first peoples*. Rochester, VT: Healing Arts Press.

OED Online. (n.d.). *Oxford English Dictionary*. Retrieved February 21, 2020, from https://www-oed-com.qe2a-proxy.mun.ca/view/Entry/196665?redirectedFrom=system#eid

Radjou, N. (2020, May 20). *NaviRadjou*. Retrieved from NaviRadjou: Uplifter, Catalyzer, Connector: http://naviradjou.com/about/

Index

P. Cornish, *Stepped Care 2.0: A Paradigm Shift in Mental Health*,
https://doi.org/10.1007/978-3-030-48055-4

Printed in Dunstable, United Kingdom

649932c4-8818-4b60-9731-cd9d0c0414feR01